☑ **W9-CTA-641**

Crossing Boundaries and Developing Alliances Through Group Work

Jocelyn Lindsay
Daniel Turcotte
Estelle Hopmeyer
Editors

ERRATUM

This booklet contains the corrected text for the section
appearing on pages 56-57.
The publisher apologizes for any inconvenience caused
by the omission of text in the original printing.

The Haworth Press®
The Haworth Press, Inc.
10 Alice Street, Binghamton, New York 13904-1580 USA

HOW SHOULD WE RESPOND?

I think we have a problem with Anglo-American traditions. At root they are competitive and individualistic and in conflict with what we believe in. However, Brown (1996) identifies three key considerations for the future of group work: values, practise-based model building, and sustaining group work and group workers into the millennium (p. 90). What I would like to propose now is a practical reassertion of group work that can encompass these considerations.

A recent briefing by the National Institute for Social Work (1996) in Britain highlights that a major cornerstone for social policy, and a challenge for social work in the new enlarging Europe, is the fight against social exclusion. It argues that the challenge of reducing social exclusion demands new approaches to individuals and groups currently denied access to employment or services.

In this context we need to return to the historical connection between group work and equality and democracy. In my work with colleagues in Europe, east and west, I am inspired when I discern in other countries and cultures where mass unemployment, demographic changes, and the apparent inability of governments to sustain their welfare provision have created various forms of social exclusion that conscious efforts are being made to reframe welfare services in ways that enhance an inclusive group-orientated approach. In contrast, in the United Kingdom, we barely have begun to address the role of social workers as agents in the fight against social exclusion and the development of models of practise that can incorporate a broader focus.

The challenge of social exclusion demands that we take account of what we have come to know about the systematic oppression of excluded groups, about antidiscriminatory practise, and about empowerment. In this context, the fundamentals of group work reassert their significance. This is because the group can be

- a source of immediate support, of friendship;
- a place to recognise shared experiences and the value of these;
- a way of breaking down isolation and loneliness;
- the source of a different perspective on personal problems; and
- a place to experience power over personal situations with the capacity to change and have an effect on these. (Butler and Wintram, 1991, p. 77)

Also, beyond these foundations, "in a group there is a better chance of addressing the inseparability of private troubles and public issues" (Breton, 1994, p. 31). Even though matters may surface as private troubles, in groups these private troubles soon become shared issues, providing the ground for the *analysis* of their structural sources and for collective *action* to bring about change (Mullender and Ward, 1991).

To illustrate what is possible, if the fundamentals are in place, I will conclude with group work examples from arguably some of the least promising areas of social work practise.

Butler (1994) writes about a group for women whose children are adjudged by social services as at risk of significant harm from their parents. She explores how the "facilitation" style of group work engendered an atmosphere of equality, enabling the women "to explore the humour, sadness and strains of family life and no longer remain silent about these" (p. 178). Central to the group agenda emerged structural dilemmas facing members: Women's sexuality and relationships with male partners were entangled with the processes of racism and the difficulties of bringing up mixed-parentage children. Faced with relentless hardships, the women easily identified the politics of poverty. Unpacking structural and individual issues was critical to these women's empowerment and the creation of their own solutions to the threats and dilemmas they faced (Butler, 1994, p. 163).

In the completely different setting of a young offenders' penal institution, Badham (1989) and colleagues worked with the inmates to develop a through-care service that the young men would see as useful and relevant by enabling them to raise issues and complaints within the institution and to prepare themselves for release. The workers sought to draw out of the young men, and to provide opportunities for them to learn, skills and knowledge that would help them survive both "inside" and after release. Confronting racist and sexist attitudes was part of this, and the worker team included women and black workers. The young men controlled the group's programme, producing, amidst wide-ranging discussions, advice booklets and arranging speakers on welfare rights, housing, parole, and temporary release. For invited speakers, including the governor, the group prepared their briefs, organised invitations, and devised questions so that they acquired the information they wanted. The governor acknowledged the value of the forum and saw in this different context hitherto unrecognised capacities in these inmates. One young man said on leaving the group, "It made you feel as though you *can* do something with your life while you are inside" (Badham, 1989, p. 35).

This then is the shape of a group work practise designed to tackle the processes of exclusion. Such group work is at its heart democratic and empowering; such group work has a place at the heart of democracy and empowerment. Of course, we must not be complacent nor uncritical, but, within group work, there are fundamentals which are sound, of which we can be proud, and which we must strive to recapture and reown.

Jocelyn Lindsay
Daniel Turcotte
Estelle Hopmeyer
Editors

Crossing Boundaries and Developing Alliances Through Group Work

Pre-publication
REVIEWS,
COMMENTARIES,
EVALUATIONS . . .

"**C**rossing Boundaries and Developing Alliances Through Group Work provides the reader with a series of excellent papers from the 19th Annual Symposium of the Association for the Advancement of Social Work with Groups, an international organization. Each chapter of the book, from Paul Taylor's insistence that groups recognize and be sensitive to cultural and national boundaries to Lawrence Shulman's complex analysis of the many boundaries crossed in working with persons with AIDS, underscores the integral aspect of a group worker's journey in establishing alliances on many levels.

Each author has a different approach, theoretically or practically, to approaching a group work practice, yet all emphasize a community of people engaged in mutual understanding and help within a context of multicultural understanding. The book would be a useful addition to a course on social group work as well as a course on cross-cultural social work.

It is rewarding to see in print a selection of what comprised a most exciting symposium that was full of hope and good will. In these difficult times, social group work provides a way for people to reach out across borders and dialogue toward more understanding. Read this book and enjoy."

Janice Andrews, PhD
Professor, School of Social Work,
University of St. Thomas,
St. Paul, MN

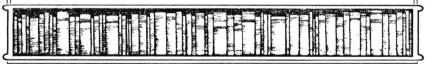

More pre-publication
REVIEWS, COMMENTARIES, EVALUATIONS . . .

"*Crossing Boundaries and Developing Alliances Through Group Work* illustrates the breadth and depth of group work and highlights the central gift group work brings to the profession: enabling people to transcend personal, cultural, and geographic isolation to give and receive mutual aid. The chapters address global and local concerns and provide insight into group work practice in its many dimensions. Group workers in direct practice in local communities, educators working to enhance students' learning opportunities in the classroom and beyond, and those working at the international level will find creative and challenging ideas in this compilation. The editors have done a superb job in selecting and presenting these articles and have provided a significant service to the profession. This collection is a welcome addition to the literature on group work."

Diane Haslett, PhD, ACSW
*Associate Professor
and BASW Program Coordinator,
University of Maine School of Social Work,
Orono, ME*

"The metaphor, crossing borders, that underlies the chapters in this collection hint at the excitement and difficulties incorporated in approaching a border. Both the desire to cross and the inherent demands to make connections on the other side create opportunities to advance practice. Crossing may be easier than maintaining the practices of the old side and melding them with the new. The eleven chapters take us into new territory, hold on to the familiar territory unique to our practice, and raise the gate for the search for the universality of group work.

The reader will find that borders can be crossed and alignments made with Asian women, mentally ill parents, and adoptive families, among others, if we are able to recognize that the walls at the borders may be scaled, or are even illusionary. Unique practice solutions are presented to deal with problems presented by group members and workers. The book provides new insights for practice in a range of contexts, and illustrates the process of group work with persons having diverse world views."

Paul Abels, PhD
*Professor Emeritus,
Department of Social Work,
California State University,
Long Beach*

More pre-publication
REVIEWS, COMMENTARIES, EVALUATIONS . . .

"**C**rossing Boundaries and Developing Alliances Through Group Work is a compilation of eleven articles presented at the 19th AASWG symposium. International and cross-cultural in perspective, this book provides a forum in which social work researchers and clinicians from around the world discuss the evolution of updated methods and practices of group work. Issues on group dynamics, working with people from all strata of society, and technological changes are discussed in this well-organized collection. The debate on sensitive topics include, but are not limited to: families involved with organ donation; mutual aid group for male sex offenders; working with families who experienced failed adoptions; and group interventions with seriously mentally ill parents.

This book also provides useful information about effective group facilitation that will be of interest to social work students and field instructors. Focusing on social work internship, Ellen Sue Mesbur and Joanne Gumpert, Sue Burrus, and John M. Duffy have respectively presented two delightful papers with ingenious and creative structures and processes that can be used in response to increasingly complex and critical needs due to social, economic, and political changes. The poem, 'Making a River,' and quotes in Chapter 6 help with the perspective and reality of students in the field. *Crossing Boundaries and Developing Alliances Through Group Work* identifies reliable approaches and suggests future directives. This can be classified as a guide and is highly recommended for all those involved in the delivery of social services."

Denise Nerette, LCSW
Faculty Field Instructor,
Barry University School of Social Work

The Haworth Press®
New York • London • Oxford

Crossing Boundaries and Developing Alliances Through Group Work

THE HAWORTH PRESS
Titles of Related Interest

Capturing the Power of Diversity edited by Marvin D. Feit, John H. Ramey, John S. Wodarski, and Aaron R. Mann

Social Group Work Today and Tomorrow: Moving from Theory to Advanced Training and Practice edited by Benj. L. Stempler and Marilyn Glass with Christine M. Savinelli

Group Work Practice in a Troubled Society: Problems and Opportunities edited by Roselle Kurland and Robert Salmon

Voices from the Field: Group Work Responds edited by Harvey Bertcher, Linda Farris Kurtz, and Alice Lamont

Strengthening Resiliency Through Group Work edited by Timothy B. Kelly, Toby Berman-Rossi, and Susanne Palomob

Social Work with Groups: Mining the Gold edited by Sue Henry, Jean East, and Cathryne Schmitz

Crossing Boundaries and Developing Alliances Through Group Work

Jocelyn Lindsay
Daniel Turcotte
Estelle Hopmeyer
Editors

The Haworth Press®
New York • London • Oxford

The Haworth Press, Inc., 10 Alice Street, Binghamton, NY 13904-1580.

PUBLISHER'S NOTE
Identities and circumstances of some individuals discussed in this book have been changed to protect confidentiality.

Chapters 1, 2, and 3 appeared previously in the French-language journal *Service Social* 46(2-3), 1997, edited by René Auclair, Jocelyn Lindsay, and Daniel Turcotte.

Cover design by Lora Wiggins.

Library of Congress Cataloging-in-Publication Data

Crossing boundaries and developing alliances through group work / Jocelyn Lindsay, Daniel Turcotte, Estelle Hopmeyer, editors.
    p. cm.
    Includes bibliographical references and index.
    ISBN 0-7890-1849-7 (hard : alk. paper)—ISBN 0-7890-1850-0 (soft : alk. paper)
    1. Social service—Teamwork. 2. Social service—Technological innovations. 3. Multicultural-ism. I. Lindsay, Jocelyn, 1944- II. Turcotte, Daniel, 1952- III. Hopmeyer, Estelle.

HV41.C763 2004
361.4—dc21
                                                                    2003001534

CONTENTS

About the Editors   ix

Contributors   xi

Acknowledgments   xv

**Introduction. Beyond Our Frontiers: The Development
of Alliances Through Group Work**   1
    Jocelyn Lindsay
    Daniel Turcotte
    Estelle Hopmeyer

**Chapter 1. Towards an International Development
of Group Work: Establishing Cultural and Linguistic
Border Crossings**   5
    Paul Taylor

Introduction   5
Internationalising Group Work   8
Arriving at the Group Work Frontier   14
The Cross-National Encounter   17
From "Inter"- to "Trans"-Cultural   19

**Chapter 2. Crossing Boundaries: Group Work
with Persons with AIDS in Early Recovery
from Substance Abuse**   27
    Lawrence Shulman

Literature Review   29
The Work   32
The Authority Theme   35
The Intimacy Theme: Helping Yourself by Helping Others   37
Conclusion   51

Chapter 3. Where Has Real Group Work Gone?
Reasserting the Fundamentals   **53**
David Ward

What Has Happened to Group Work?   54
How Should We Respond?   56

Chapter 4. Group Field Consulting: Building
a Learning Community   **59**
Ellen Sue Mesbur

Introduction   59
Development of Supervision and Field Instruction
    in Social Work   60
The Group Field-Consulting Model   64
Conclusions   68
Appendix: Field-Consulting Methodology
    and Outcomes   70

Chapter 5. Night of the Tortured Souls: Integration
of Group Therapy and Mutual Aid for Treated
Male Sex Offenders   **75**
Dennis Kimberley
Louise Osmond

Integrating Continued Therapy with Supervised
    Mutual Aid   75
A Philosophy of Treating and Supporting the Treated   79
Group Practice in Integrating Therapy and Mutual Aid
    with Treated Sex Offenders   83
Conclusion   94

Chapter 6. Pushing the Boundary and Coming
Full Circle: A Contemporary Role for Social
Group Work in Service Education   **99**
Joanne Gumpert
Sue Burrus
John M. Duffy

Literature Review   100
The Field Placement   104
Effects of the Group Work Intervention   107

Future Directions   111
Appendix: Levels of Transcendence Identified in Group
    Interaction   112

**Chapter 7. The Use of Teleconferencing Focus Groups
with Families Involved in Organ Donation:
Dealing with Sensitive Topics**   **115**
        Sandra Regan

Why Teleconferencing Focus Groups?   115
Dealing with Sensitive Topics   117
Reactivity in the Screener Questionnaire   119
Motivation of the Participants   122
Moderators' Self-Disclosure and Credibility   123
Group Members' Self-Disclosure   126
Normalisation of Emotions   127
Legitimisation of Participants' Comments   128
Building on Preparation and Beginning the Focus Group   129
Conclusion   130

**Chapter 8. Using Groups for Research and Action:
The Asian Mothers' Support Project**   **133**
        Lorraine Gutiérrez
        Izumi Sakamoto
        Tom Morson

The North Campus Outreach Project   134
A Program and a Process for Change   136
Programming   139
Survey and Program Data   140
Results   141
Synergy Through Groups   142
Summary   144

**Chapter 9. Families for Reunification: A Mediating
Group Model for Birth Parent Self-Assessment**   **147**
        Michael W. Wagner

Partners in the Plan   147
Program Development   149
Program Design   152

Analysis   157
Conclusion   161
Appendix: Families for Reunification—Partners
   in the Plan, Final Assessment   162

**Chapter 10. Efficacy of Group Interventions
with Seriously Mentally Ill Parents:
A Literature Review**   **167**
   Gordon MacDonald

Introduction   167
Definition of a Group   168
The Population   170
Seriously Mentally Ill Parents and Group Intervention   174
Implications   181
Conclusion   187

**Chapter 11. Post–Legal Adoption Treatment Groups:
Intervening with Families Who Experience Failed
Adoptions**   **193**
   Karen V. Harper-Dorton

Introduction   193
Adoption Disruption/Dissolution: Definitions
   and Overview   194
Demographics of the Population Studied   196
The Importance of Post–Legal Adoption Intervention   197
Group Services   198
Program Design   199
Curriculum   199
Outcome and Follow-Up   204
Conclusions   206

Index   **209**

ABOUT THE EDITORS

Jocelyn Lindsay, PhD, is Professor and Director, School of Social Work, Laval University in Quebec City, Canada, where he teaches courses in group work intervention, theories of social work with groups, social prevention, men's issues, and social work and family violence. Dr. Lindsay's research interests focus on group processes, evaluation of intervention, husband-wife violence, and professional ethics.

Daniel Turcotte, PhD, is Professor and Director of the Master Program, School of Social Work, Laval University in Quebec City, Canada, where he teaches courses on group work at the undergraduate level and on qualitative research and social support at the graduate level. Dr. Turcotte's research interests focus on families and children with a special emphasis on program evaluation.

Estelle Hopmeyer, MSW, is Professor and Director of the Master Program, School of Social Work, Laval University in Quebec City, Canada, where she teaches courses in group work at the undergraduate and graduate levels, and a Master's course in loss and bereavement. Ms. Hopmeyer's research interests focus on loss and bereavement, suicide, AIDS, disenfranchised grief, and end-of-life concerns. She is Coordinator of the McGill Center for Loss and Bereavement, which provides free support groups to the Montreal community.

CONTRIBUTORS

Sue Burrus, MSW, LSW, Community Relations Coordinator, Washington State Association of Court Appointed Special Advocate Program, Seattle, Washington.

John M. Duffy, MSW, LSW, Intensive Outpatient Group Worker, New Concepts Treatment Group, Hallstead, Pennsylvania.

Joanne Gumpert, DSW, Associate Professor, School of Social Work, Marywood University, Scranton, Pennsylvania.

Lorraine Gutiérrez, PhD, Professor, University of Michigan School of Social Work, Ann Arbor, Michigan.

Karen V. Harper-Dorton, PhD, Professor, School of Applied Social Sciences, West Virginia University, Morgantown, West Virginia.

Dennis Kimberley, PhD, RSW, Professor, School of Social Work, Memorial University of Newfoundland, St. John's, Newfoundland, Canada.

Gordon MacDonald, Doctoral Student, Faculty of Social Work, University of Toronto, Toronto, Ontario, Canada.

Ellen Sue Mesbur, MSW, EdD, Director, School of Social Work, Renison College, University of Waterloo, Waterloo, Ontario, Canada.

Tom Morson, MSW, ACSW, Counseling and Psychological Services, University of Michigan, Ann Arbor, Michigan.

Louise Osmond, MSW, RSW, Clinical Social Worker and Consultant, Advanced Therapy and Consulting Services, St. John's, Newfoundland, Canada.

Sandra Regan, PhD, Senior Lecturer, School of Social Work, University of New South Wales, Sydney, Australia.

Izumi Sakamoto, MSW, PhD, Assistant Professor, Faculty of Social Work, University of Toronto, Toronto, Ontario, Canada.

Lawrence Shulman, MSW, EdD, Professor and Dean, School of Social Work, State University of New York at Buffalo.

Paul Taylor, Institut Supérieur de Formation Permanente, Université François Rabelais, Tours, France.

Michael W. Wagner, MSW, Administrative Supervisor, Intake Unit, The Children's Aid Society, New York, New York.

David Ward, LLB, MA, Professor, Department of Social and Community Studies, School of Health and Applied Social Sciences, De Montfort University, Leicester, England.

Bonnie J. Engelhardt, Needham, MA
Mary Pender Greene, Brooklyn, NY
Joanne Gumpert, Scranton, PA
Carolyn Knight, Westminster, MD
Andrew Malekoff, Long Beach, NY
Ellen Sue Mesbur, Toronto, Ontario, Canada

- **Chapter Representatives:**

California—Joan K. Parry, Vista, CA
Connecticut—Susan Lalone, Danvers, MA
Florida—David F. Fike, Miami Shores, FL
Georgia—Benjamin L. Stempler, Lawrenceville, GA
Germany—Ingrun Masanek, Norden, Germany
Kentucky—Mary Jean Kellett, Louisville, KY
Long Island—Susan G. Rosner, Jericho, NY
Massachusetts—Jerry S. Jacobs, Needham, MA
Minnesota—Carol Kuechler, St. Paul, MN
New Jersey—Lisa Dribbon, Flemington, NJ
New York—Urania E. Glassman, New York, NY
Ohio—Christine A. Dusek-Myers, Cleveland, OH
Toronto—Nancy E. Sullivan, Toronto, Canada

Counsel: Steve Kraft, Attorney-at-Law, Grand Forks, ND

Acknowledgments

The following people helped to plan and manage the nineteenth annual symposium of the Association for the Advancement of Social Work with Groups: Marie Berlinguet, retired social worker and administrator; Isabelle Côté, Sainte-Foy/Sillery Community Health Center; Estelle Hopmeyer, McGill University School of Social Work; Nataly Jacques, Beauport Association of Community Services; Jocelyn Lindsay, Laval University School of Social Work; Daniel Turcotte, Laval University School of Social Work; and Jean-François Vézina, Quebec Resource for Violent Men.

The School of Social Work, Faculty of Social Sciences, Laval University, was the sponsor of the XIX Annual Symposium of the AASWG, with the participation of many organizations, agencies, and services as well as the support of many individuals.

We are pleased to acknowledge with gratitude the grants provided by the Social Sciences and Humanities Research Council of Canada, the Simone Paré Foundation, and the Professional Order of Social Workers of the province of Quebec.

The editors would like to thank the numerous volunteers who worked countless hours, as well as the presenters, session chairpersons, participants, and staff of the Hilton Hotel for making this symposium a meaningful and enjoyable experience.

A special note of appreciation must also be given to John Ramey, whose advice was invaluable in the planning process.

Introduction

Beyond Our Frontiers:
The Development of Alliances
Through Group Work

Jocelyn Lindsay
Daniel Turcotte
Estelle Hopmeyer

This title stems from the theme of the nineteenth annual symposium of the Association for the Advancement of Social Work with Groups, which was held in Québec City October 23-29, 1997. On this occasion, more than 400 people from thirteen countries crossed their frontiers and were united during these four days to discuss social work with groups in large group forums, workshops, special presentations, groups sessions with experts, as well as in their exchanges with other delegates. In this text, we will elaborate on the meaning of and reasons for this symposium theme and introduce the content of the symposium proceedings.

Crossing frontiers and establishing alliances is as much an integral part of the group worker's life as the development of mutual help between people is the foundation of social work with groups. Within the development of what is to become pertinent tools for social work practice, we must, at times, cross frontiers and barriers as they arise. If we look at this situation from another perspective, we can observe that particular conditions (on the technological, economic, and social planes) create contexts for new problems to emerge that must be resolved. In many instances, these contexts also provide numerous possibilities to redefine our professional field.

The creation of alliances is an important way to reduce the limits that we are confronted by and permits us to make valuable contributions toward a more promising future. Given this, how can we actual-ize the development of alliances using group work's essential charac-teristics as part of this promising future? Without trying to exhaustively describe the different facets of this question, we can mention certain strategies whereby social workers regularly operationalize the development of such alliances. These strategies were, in fact, the subject of many of the symposium presentations.

The first aspect touches the multicultural dimension of our work, which is an essential element that must be taken into consideration in order to overcome some of the isolation that confronts many of the populations with whom we work. The second aspect concerns the ben-eficial effects of the junction between research and intervention. How can social work with groups converge with other fields of knowledge (i.e., the arts, music, and drama), or with other intervention theories, to contribute to a more efficient intervention methodology? On an or-ganizational level, the partnership between research teams and the agencies that dispense services can be equally beneficial for both parties. With regard to education and training, field placements constitute the major element in the training of social work with groups, and they re-quire collaboration between schools and practice settings. In the ac-tual development of social work with groups, the schools give their students an advantage when they collaborate with these organizations because this partnership assures a greater quality of education. The arrival of new technologies, such as teleconferencing and the Inter-net, make it possible to hold discussions and exchange ideas, an ad-vantage that was virtually nonexistent or impossible a decade ago. An additional form of alliance that can be experienced by those workers who are involved in group intervention is the complementary contri-butions and benefits of combining, "mixing and matching," or alter-nating between different intervention methodologies within the field of social work to produce a more effective intervention strategy.

We would like to introduce the chapters that have been selected to represent these proceedings by providing a brief description of their various focuses and content. The first three texts were presented in large group forums and are in direct relation to the symposium theme. Paul Taylor's lecture began with the question "How can we create an educative praxis of social group work, at an international level, com-mitted to the collective human struggle for a radically more just soci-ety, while fully respecting the notion of difference and cultural identity in any given group?" In this presentation, Taylor underlines the necessity for international group work development to begin with, and continually include, a fundamental understanding of national identity, of cultural belonging, and the influence of these factors on the groups' dynamics. In another forum presentation, Lawrence Shulman uses as an illustration a project in which he co-led a group of persons with AIDS in early recovery from substance abuse. He develops the idea of crossing boundaries and developing alliances on a number of levels: academic and community agencies, research and practice, social work and substance abuse counseling, mutual aid and twelve-step models, etc. David Ward proposes to examine what is happening to group work in Great Britain; he argues that we need to return to the historical connection between group work and equality and democracy to tackle the processes of exclusion.

Despite the seemingly great variation in the next five chapters, a common element unites each of them to the others. Each of the authors associates group work with other theoretical frames of reference or methodologies as a means by which to provide a greater quality of service to those being assisted by the various interventions. An interest in building a learning community is portrayed by Ellen Sue Mesbur's work, where she illustrates the connection between social group work tools and adult learning principles. Group field consultation is viewed as a medium for the development of mutual assistance among students, field instructors, and faculty field consultants. Dennis Kimberley and Louise Osmond describe a pilot project to treat male sex offenders, in which group therapy based on psychoeducational components is integrated with mutual assistance to create a comprehensive community-based treatment model. Joanne Gumpert, Sue Burrus, and John M. Duffy discuss a cooperative arrangement where graduate social work students facilitate group sessions for undergraduate students participating in spring break volunteer service trips. With this particular example, social group work is integrated with in-service learning. Students are placed within a particular community service setting and must later analyze the experience within an academic framework. In the next chapter, Sandra Regan explores the use of time-limited teleconferencing focus groups with families previously involved in organ donations. Although the individuals were united for a needs assessment and not group counseling, it remains a useful example of the use of group work skills in conjunction with focus group methodology in order to create a favorable environment for the discussion of sensitive matters. The chapter presented by Lorraine Gutiérrez, Izumi Sakamoto, and Tom Morson gives information on an action research project developed to address the needs of international students and their families. Focus groups, task groups, educational and mutual assistance/self-help groups provide an arena for bringing together different voices required for a truly multicultural effort.

The last three chapters in these proceedings place importance on the use of group work when dealing with specific questions. The alliances that are discussed in these chapters are those which occur within the group and also between the group members and people in their immediate environment. Michael W. Wagner describes a group designed to assist and support birth families in developing a self-assessment of strengths and needs for family reunification (within an agency context devoted to a "strengths perspective" approach). Gordon MacDonald's chapter is a review of the literature regarding the efficacy of group interventions with parents who have a serious mental illness. It provides a level of awareness regarding the quantity, quality, and effectiveness of group modalities. Karen V. Harper-Dorton notes the need to develop post–legal adoption group treatment services for families at risk of adoption disruption. Group intervention is presented as a model of choice for intervening with adopted children and their parents at risk of ending their adoptions and terminating family relationships due to very troubled and emotionally damaging family dynamics.

Chapter 1

Towards an International Development of Group Work: Establishing Cultural and Linguistic Border Crossings

Paul Taylor

INTRODUCTION

The problem really is the title. Where is the *international* supposed to go? The international development of group work, or the development of international group work? If it is the latter, we should probably be talking more about cross-cultural group work. If it is to be the former, we are not really talking about group work but about the sociopolitical context in which it might take place. In either case, who is doing the (group) work, and who is supposed to be doing the development?

To put the question like that is not just an easy way to find an introduction to this session. In a very real sense, if we are clearer about the question and certainly if we have the beginnings of an answer by the end of this international symposium, we shall indeed know that we have moved *towards* new dimensions in group work.

There are two main reasons why even defining the question is difficult. The first is that almost every aspect of our daily lives, personal and professional, is becoming more and more subject to the forces of *mondialisation* or *globalisation.* We are beginning, on the one hand, to understand how the "Web," Inter-, Extra-, Supra- (to take the most powerful of the images of the new technologies), reduces our mental "living space." Distance is just an e-mail away, information and communication are available around the clock and around the globe. Like it or not, knowingly or not, we are all now caught in the Net; we have become intergalactic surfers, intercontinental correspondents, and international shoppers.

5

Far from being a humanising or idealising *écoumène*,[1] this new social order is a very real mega-economy. The processes of mondialisation are essentially economic, driven by the multinationals and the players of the global stock market and fueled by an unshakable belief in the doctrine that free-exchangism means the right to take profits anywhere, at any time, from anybody. The old, multicolored political maps of Europe, the Far East, and the Americas are giving way to new maps of supranational trading unions and alliances, identified as "zones" for the exclusive use of the dollar, the ECU, or the yen.

This homogenisation of culture, from the standardisation even architecturally of nearly all our large towns, to the ubiquitous Macdo, jeans uniform, and the linguistic hegemony of English, is a phenomenon overdetermined[2] by economics. To understand many of these developments, we need to begin by appreciating the first laws of modern economics.

That might be difficult enough to relate directly to group work, but the second reason why our original question poses problems is that there is an enormous, and at times equally frightening, countermovement in revolt against this imposed universalism. It almost seems to be the case that the more we globalise, the more we need to localise. In almost every country in the world, there is a revival of nationalism and regionalism: the claims of the Indian nations in North and South America; South Timor; the Basque country; Corsica; Macedonia; the Kurds; the proposals for devolved parliaments in Scotland and Wales; the continuing troubles in Ireland; the demands for a free Palestine; Bosnia; Malaysia; even Quebec where we are today. The list is long and often marked by conflict, terrorism, and counteroppression.

This sense of national identity is complex, identifying a community of interest founded on a shared history, specific cultural values, religious allegiances, ethnic purity, territorial claims to land or sea, or identifiable language zones. People want to reassert their individuality, their identity, their right not to be lost, individually or collectively, in the anonymous, depersonalised macroworld where their only worth is economic.

At one level that is perfectly understandable, but we need to ask, "How do we understand it?" It is an important fact that, as yet, this movement towards nationalism remains largely undertheorised. Historians have *described* the rise and fall of Nazism, but we still do not generally understand the relationship that existed between Hitler, the Third Reich, and the German people. Politicians have deplored the obscenity of ethnic purification in Bosnia and Rwanda, and humanitarian aid has rushed to stem the tide of human suffering, but we still do not understand the underlying causes. Anthropologists and sociologists have identified some of the factors of different, conflicting "nationalisms." But what are the dominant theories that underpin these statements of fact? Without a sound theoretical base, there is always a danger that we will find a good answer, but to the wrong question.

It may be one of the outcomes of this symposium that practitioners of group work begin to explore together a program of research-action within their differing practices to begin to address this fundamental problem. It may seem that we are straying a long way from the day-to-day practise of group work into some kind of indulgent, academic theorising. Let me give one brief example of the need to research together.

One of the key questions to be addressed is that of the *state*. We cannot begin to develop international group work without asking ourselves, "What do we mean by *international?*" What is the relationship between *state* and *nation?* Many of the different nationalist movements seem intent on reinventing the idea of the *nation-state* that made a jigsaw of kingdoms and principalities across Europe in the fifteenth and sixteenth centuries. The "Northern League" in Italy is a typical example. Or the debate in France about immigration controls that effectively define citizenship exclusively in terms of the principles of the Revolution and the privileged relationship between the *citoyen* and *la République française*. Or, again, the wider debate in Europe claiming first a common currency and then a single currency hinges on two different visions of Europe: one is a multiplex federation of nation-states, the other a simplex, supranational union.

We may well want to reinvent the nation-state, but, equally, we cannot at the same time disinvent the more modern idea of the *welfare state*. All countries now seem to agree, following a generalised principle of "social subsidiarity," that the state should take on certain responsibilities that surpass the means or the competencies of its individual citizens, for example, social security, social assistance, medicare, pensions and assurance, and protection for workers as well as the young, the elderly, or the handicapped. However, as we know as workers in our various social fields, the very essence of *welfare* is that it should be local, at least at the point of delivery. Social work itself can be defined as the institutionalised "go-between" of the state and individual need.

The final element of the problem: given the size of the social security budget, the increasing needs for long-term welfare, the noncontribution to the system because of unemployment, an increasingly aging population, and the need to sustain pension funds by juggling investment portfolios, etc., the resourcing of welfare has become, like the arms industry, another international industry. Welfare policy is delivered locally but defined globally.

So, if we were to ask in the different countries, for example, "Who is working in community care?" or "Who is working in community education?", the reply would have to be filtered by our own understanding of the state, the nation, and the community. "Community care," for example, in the United States, in France, in Greece, or in the Scandinavian countries, does not refer to the same practises, the same principles of social action, nor the same social policy. One of the invisible but very real barriers to cross-national group work in community care, to take but one example, is that workers may well deal with the same clientele, may use the same professional jargon, but do not have the same fundamental understandings about what constitutes "care in the community."

INTERNATIONALISING GROUP WORK

Where then can we begin? Happily, some of the ingredients are given: the (international) development of (international) group work (IDIG) requires

1. an understanding of "national identity";
2. an understanding of "cultural belonging"; and, therefore,
3. an understanding of how national identity and cultural belonging impact the dynamics of any given group.

My first experience of crossing group work frontiers was many years ago in West Africa where I became particularly interested in the management of crisis and the resolution of conflict in the different cultures of the Sahel while working with the International Red Cross.

This "melting pot" of good intentions was revealing: the crisis was local, due to the drought, but the conflict was more often than not European.

More recently, teaching and working in Europe, I have become interested in one particular aspect of group life, the meeting. The role and function of a "meeting" is not the same in the different European cultures: for one, it is a place for discussion; for another, it serves for the transmission of information; in another, it is the place to confirm decisions already taken. Yet each meeting has its own code and procedures, hierarchies and deviancies, and it is sometimes very difficult to learn how to behave and how to contribute (or not).

The work of Bollinger and Hofstede is as ever a valuable starting point.[3] Essentially, through very extensive interviews, they sought to identify national typologies of managerial behavior, a typology that I willingly exploit for the following reason. My working hypothesis is that social groups tend to behave in line with the dominant models of management in vogue in any given country. These initial typologies of Bollinger and Hofstede are not stereotypes that might simply massage our various national prejudices; they are typical or standardised behavior as evidenced by the interviewees themselves.

Bollinger and Hofstede[4] studied fifty-three countries and created a differential rating scale that allows comparisons to be made between different national models. Each country then has a ranking scale (1 to 53) and an individual score (normally between 0 and 110). Their research identifies four key elements on which perceptions differ considerably across national boundaries.

Relative Hierarchical Distance

How does a given society perceive the degree of inequality or distance between those who hold power and those who are subject to that power? How do they consult, delegate, value contrary opinion, take initiatives, and personalise responsibility? Using the answers to these questions to measure the continuum of power, establishing the psychological and social dynamic that exists in any given group, we can begin to calculate the relative hierarchical distance (RHD). For example, countries with a high RHD will prefer modes of communication and interaction that tend to be autocratic and paternalistic. Low RHD indicates a preference for consultative or democratic group procedures.

Latin countries tend to have a higher RHD than Germanic countries; high-technology cultures have low RHD; poorer countries, where the difference between the powerful and the powerless is evident, normally have a high RHD.

Relative Hierarchical Distance

Ranking	Country	Score
5	Mexico	81
7	Saudi Arabia	80
14	Brazil	69
16	France	68
24	Chile	63
33	Japan	54
38	United States	40
39	Canada	39
44	United Kingdom	35
52	Israel	13

Individuality

Different societies construct the continuum "society–community–family–individual" in different ways: some are far more "communal societies," while others are far more centered on the individual. The former stresses the *us:* social equality and a person's role rather than personality. The latter prefers the *me:* social difference and individuality. Obviously the processes of immigration and emigration with such groups are not the same.

Are certain cultures more cooperative or competitive? Does social change follow an evolutionary, logical, and orderly pattern without major revolutions, or does it lurch from left to right, create and change alliances, discard the useless or the incompetent?

Degree of Individuality

Ranking	Country	Score
1	United States	91
3	United Kingdom	89
4	Canada	80
11	France	71
19	Israel	54
22	Japan	46
26	Brazil	38
27	Saudi Arabia	38
32	Mexico	30
38	Chile	23

Gender

Gender roles and expectations are clearly a basic component of group work but certainly not universal. In some countries, high-status roles are automatically masculine and it is usually the male who is socially, culturally, and economically advantaged. Bollinger and Hofstede used a shorthand distinction between a "male culture" that clearly differentiates between male/female roles, and a "female culture" where there is role equality and interchangeability.

The conclusions here are stark. Male cultures tend to be competitive, status aware, product oriented, but technology dependent. Female cultures, particularly in small groups, tend to be process oriented, pay more attention to the ambiance of the group that will facilitate cooperation and exchange, are competence rather than status aware, and exploit more its human rather than its technological resources.

Gender Difference

Ranking	Country	Score
1	Japan	95
6	Mexico	69
9	United Kingdom	66
15	United States	62
23	Saudi Arabia	53
24	Canada	52
27	Brazil	49
29	Israel	47
36	France	43
46	Chile	28

Risk Taking

How do we see the future? How do we cope with change? Some groups need the support of clear rules and regulations, to curtail the scope of uncertainty, and require precise procedures, identifying who is or is not in the group, and always have some superior "court of appeal." Other groups thrive on initiative, intuition, and the freedom to change and adapt at will because they are able to take more personal risks and manage greater individual responsibility.

Some countries, like the United States, are identifiably risk cultures; others insist on high levels of control and accord high status to the "expert" or consultant, the doctor who can put all things right.

Risk Taking

Ranking	Country	Score
7	Japan	92
10	France	86
11	Chile	86
18	Mexico	82
19	Israel	81
22	Brazil	76
27	Saudi Arabia	68
42	Canada	48
43	United States	46
47	United Kingdom	35

An overview of these four cultural dimensions shows, albeit numerically, the points of resemblance and difference among the different nations/cultures (here in alphabetical order):

Country	RHD	Individuality	Gender	Risk Taking
Brazil	14	26	27	22
Canada	39	4	24	42
Chile	24	38	46	11
France	16	11	36	10
Israel	52	19	29	19
Japan	33	22	1	7
Mexico	5	32	6	18
Saudi Arabia	7	27	23	27
United Kingdom	44	3	9	47
United States	38	1	15	43

ARRIVING AT THE GROUP WORK FRONTIER

International group work is not some enormous chameleon that adapts itself to the colors of a national flag or adjusts itself mentally to the dominant culture wherever it happens to be. If this were the case, we would never know what it was we were really trying to achieve. No, group work is rather a knot of ideologies, practises, and processes of communication and social interaction related to the given society which produces it and which, in turn, it reproduces. International group work represents a change in scale and therefore in complexity, but not in fundamentals.

What is needed is not simply to describe national differences but to construct a framework of analysis that will enable us to go further. Although it is always interesting to explore how to behave in a cross-cultural situation, our primary task is to discover *where* this situation might be. In other words, what happens to the idea of "group work" when we add the adjective "international"? The objective of creating alliances that this symposium has set itself is in fact more a response to the question *where* than to the question *how*.

The analytical framework that I am proposing here presents a kind of mapping of the terrain. The four strands of our group work knot reveal the process that has become known classically, since Tuckman, as a process of forming–storming–norming–performing.[5] (Many other models of group development would suit equally well, depending on whether we wanted to put the emphasis on the early stages of group life, the overall process, or its productivity.) If we then cross these strands with our four lines of critical inquiry (hierarchy, individuality, gender, and risk taking) we can produce a matrix that poses some serious but very fascinating questions.

I have presented the matrix as a "magic square" in order to insist symbolically on the interrelation among all the elements (see Figure 1.1).[6] In all directions the sum of the problem is the same, but we are able to approach it from widely differing, even contradictory, angles. Because the magic square is arbitrary—you can start from any point with any number—there is no intended hierarchy of values. I aim only to create a device that will first identify different perspectives and core questions and then allow us to compare and contrast what we might find at the various intersections. Obviously each intersection, each synaptic point (which we can refer to by its number), repre-

	Forming	Storming	Norming	Performing
Hierarchical distance	7	12	1	14
Individuality	2	13	8.	11
Gender	16	3	10	5
Risk taking	9	6	15	4

FIGURE 1.1. Magic Square Matrix

sents a site where, potentially, group workers might intervene. These are our imaginary observation points along the frontier.

Identifying the Frontiers of International Group Work

We can use the matrix to juggle an enormous number of ideas, values, institutions, cultures, and practises. There are no "correct" answers, but the use of the matrix at least helps us to locate ourselves in the debate. This is important because we have to come to terms with the fact that, at the point of intercultural meeting, not all the participants are necessarily crossing the same frontier. Obviously, we need some examples.

Point 2: The Need to Be Polite

In the early stages of group life—the first meetings, milling around, getting to know one another—almost all cultures work within a framework of politeness, but simply being polite is not enough. How do you intend to be polite? Taking the principle that no interpersonal encounter is "faceless" (and the concept of "face" is clearly critical here), we can identify three differing processes of politeness, each operating within a dual dynamic of *distance* and *power.*[7]

The first is a *deference* process, whereby group members treat one another with a high degree of respect (using formal titles, *vous/Usted* or an equivalent), while maintaining their distance. As a formula, we could describe it as $-P+D$: such a behavioral pattern is normal in many Far Eastern or South American cultures.

The second is a *solidarity* process, expressing equality but implying that there is already a close, personal relationship or the intention to create one: $-P-D$, a pattern that one sees frequently within a North American professional and business culture. The third reflects a hierarchical politeness very conscious of the inequality of status and power: $+P$ and the dynamic marked by either $-D$ or $+D$. Important in these situations is that the politeness procedure is symmetrical, but this is obviously difficult to attain in a meeting between high RHD cultures and, for example, high individuality cultures.

Point 12: Being Selfish/Self-Centered

This year I made a rare visit to London with a group of French adult educators to participate in a cross-cultural seminar. During one of the initial, plenary discussions in which we were preparing the program, one of the British students, who was supposed to be "hosting" the session, suddenly said, "But I don't see how my learning needs are going to be met. What I am looking for is . . ." The group was shocked, almost unable to respond except by accommodating her wishes. But where does *self-centered learning* fit into the cultural construction of a group, given the interplay between RHD and individuality, especially in the early stages of group life? The student obviously thought she was negotiating; many others felt she was being insensitively provocative.

Point 5: A Women-Only Group?

Coming from a culture where it is quite normal for a group of women to work together, I have frequently tried to understand why French students and social workers have always refused this option. Not surprising, many men are against the idea in principle, but more surprising is the fact that many women equally see no point in "excluding men" from the group.

This is effectively the obverse of the syndrome that I observed when a British colleague came to our university. I explained some of the cultural dynamics of the distinctive French education system. "I can tolerate all that" she said but added, "anything except sexism." The problem, however, is not one of tolerance. The problem is to be clear about what constitutes sexism or, even more difficult, what constitutes antisexism in differing cultures.

THE CROSS-NATIONAL ENCOUNTER

Given the different levels at which we operate professionally in groups, it would be important to look more closely at the complexity of a cross-national encounter. We can assume that we are talking here about contacts that are essentially interpersonal rather than inter-institutional. Transnational *organisational* or *political* contacts require a different analysis, but even within group work these contacts are inevitably pluridimensional.

Contact between a group worker and his or her group (G) with the other culture/nation (OC/N) may be

- through meeting and incorporating into the group an individual from an OC/N (OC/N1);
- through meeting and associating with an OC/N group (OC/N2);
- through meeting an individual or a group who represents, not a single individual or individuals, but the institutions of the culture/nation, for example, a representative of the education or welfare system, the police, civic or church authorities, or a national team (OC/N3).

Conversely, the group worker and his or her group may be the ones being incorporated into the OC/N. In this sense, the home group culture/nation (HG) has three ways of encountering the OC/N:

- one individual finds himself or herself in a "foreign" group (HG1);
- the home group is working in a foreign culture (HG2);

- the home group or the individuals represent not the group or themselves but the home culture/nation or its institutions (HG3).

For example, some of the foreign participants in this symposium who have come here out of personal interest and in an individual capacity may well see themselves as HG1 but could easily be treated as OC/N3. What will happen in the small group sessions? Will the dominant English-speaking group (HG2) actually behave more like OC/N2? How will we decide the ambiance and the rules of our own international encounter?

No international or intercultural encounter is neutral. Even if we proclaim *Vive la différence!* or subscribe to a liberalism that asserts "equality through difference," we cannot escape the fact that, to the degree that one culture/nation seeks to dominate the other or cedes place to the other on account of some real or imagined attribute, positive or negative, the interpretation of the encounter will be radically different.

We know enough about the complexity of changes in the content of interaction in small groups composed of dyads and triads not to rush too quickly into the dimension of a truly *multi*national encounter. Let us first illustrate the point by looking at the encounter *à deux*. Culture or nation A may dominate or seek to dominate B, so their encounter takes place in an environment of Ab. B may dominate or seek to dominate A, hence a quite different encounter aB. Or A and B might meet on the basis of either equal status or equal power, AB. Accepting that, we can plot perceived positions on a graph. Who is meeting whom? On what terms? Within what dynamics of culture-power relationships?

Look again at the visitor, and let us say she is German or French. She may see herself as an experienced field-worker abroad and enjoy working in a language and culture that is not her own. She might define herself along a line HG1–Ab. Other members of the symposium, concerned to value the "otherness" of her experience, try their best to redress the cultural disequilibrium but come to treat her as typical of German or French social work and group work practise. They react along line AB–OC/N3, as shown here:

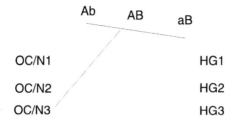

The starting point must be to accept the individual's or the group's perceived judgement of where they are in the encounter. This is another way to emphasise the importance of the two distinct views of culture that I have described as *emic* and *etic*.[8] Both views are necessarily culturocentric, in the sense that culture is one of the prime means of expressing identity and social belonging. The processes of integration, acculturation, and socialisation all converge to provide the individual, group, and community with a cultural center. We learn to belong, to center ourselves on a given way of life and on certain values, to have roots, and to recognise those who share those roots and those who do not. Culturocentrism is to the group what egocentrism is to the individual. I have to start with the fact that I am who I am if I want to ask you who you are.

The distinction between emics and etics is not new and reflects the development of ideas that have their roots in Tajfel's theory of the "we group" and the broader "insider-outsider" debate.[9] The emic view is from the inside, from the lived experience, and structured by the values inherent in the system. The etic view is from the outside and from the learned experience, basing its judgement on values exterior to the system. I think, however, we are just beginning to see its potential as a tool of transcultural and transnational group work.

FROM "INTER"- TO "TRANS"-CULTURAL

Social group work is often used as a method of social integration, individual rehabilitation, or cultural assimilation. The group is both an economic way of working, but more especially one of the best means of creating the solidarity and cohesion necessary for effective social action. Given that the problems created by unemployment, discrimination, poverty, and ill health have no respect for national boundaries, it is quite natural that group workers should look towards international settings to find responses even to very local difficulties.

We cannot escape from this dynamic between the micro and the macro. If workers think, however, only on a micro local level, they may well be able to help a certain number of individuals, but they may not be able to go beyond treating the symptoms of the problem. The distinction made by Wright Mills is important: we should not confuse what is a personal difficulty and what is essentially a social problem.[10]

If we are working with a group of unemployed or mentally ill patients, there is much to be done to create the confidence and exchange within the group that will have potentially very positive outcomes for each individual. However, if we look only at these individual horizons, we will be doing nothing to combat the social problem, unemployment, or the social factors that provoke and encourage mental illness. Very quickly, social group work ends up "blaming the victims."

One can legitimately ask the question "How much of our professional time is actually given over to working on this macro sociopolitical horizon?" But even this question presupposes that competencies necessary for working on national and international levels have already been acquired. At the extreme, we find, for example, workers involved in creative work with newly arrived immigrants, who see their work only monoculturally; they do not seek to involve themselves in relationships with the country from which the immigrants have come. Or we see postretirement groups who are not involved in the preretirement world of work, a world that cannot escape from the influences of multinationalism.

It does not follow from my appeal that health, education, poverty, employment, social security, or immigration, etc., should not be treated as parochial but as transnational issues, that I think such problems are experienced in the same way in all cultures. There are far too many other factors, economic, moral, environmental, and political, that can make the lived experience very different from one country to another. The opportunity to explore such differences is one of the exciting and most fruitful benefits of this symposium.

I am, however, proposing that the ability to work at a transnational level, as well as at a transcultural level, should be seen as a basic competency of an effective group worker. This does not require that each group worker becomes an activist on the political or economic front, but it does mean that he or she has the confidence and the competence *as a group worker* to cross national/cultural frontiers.

This is what we need to "problematise," to use one of Freire's favorite words—not to "make problems," but to visualise "as a problem." If there is no problem, then there is no solution. My basic hypothesis is that the ability to work binationally is analogous to that of being bilingual. Both are based on the processes of *translation*. This is critical because all too often the international or intercultural encounter is thought of only as a more complicated form of "A meets B in X." Schematically, we can represent the transcultural meeting as:

$$Culture\ A \to\to X \leftarrow\leftarrow Culture\ B$$

In Europe today, we can cross frontiers without passports, without customs controls, without even changing gear, so that we are even physically less aware of preparing to "meet" another nation or culture. This model, therefore, because of its simplicity, actually conceals a more complex process that reveals not just one but several cultural "meeting points." I have here adopted and greatly developed a model taken, like the emics and etics debate, from the discipline of linguistics and translation (see Figure 1.2).[11]

The actual meeting A⟷B represents the visible elements that we can observe as practise or performance. What remains hidden is the infrastructure or metastructure of interculturalism, the points 2–3–4. Any genuine intercultural encounter has to be a reciprocal movement from A through 2–3–4 to B, and from B through its own 2–3–4 back to A:

$$A \to (2 - 3 - 4) \to B : B \to (2 - 3 - 4) \to A$$

It is in these zones of 2–3–4 that the communicative competencies of interculturality lie.

If we take as an example the line 12–13–3–6 of our matrix (Figure 1.1) and look at the processes of storming and of dissent in a group, we note that groups with a high RHD express conflict and disagreement with a great deal of heat, forceful expressions, shouting, and a fair element of theatre. On the other hand, groups with a high degree of risk taking minimize overt anger and express dissent by glacial politeness, calm but cutting remarks, or insolent silence.

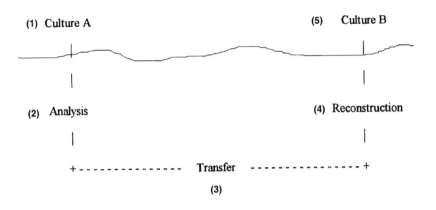

FIGURE 1.2. Constructing the Cultural Encounter

In a cross-cultural setting, both groups would have to have the capacity first of all to analyse their own behavior, values, and strategies. They would then need to transfer that understanding of what they intended to communicate into another register and reconstruct their normal response in such a way that it was meaningful to the other. This is nothing other than a normal process of translation.

Translation exposes the differences between languages as between cultures. Our analysis of it enables us to understand the strangeness of the other and the degree to which we have to adapt in order to find common ground. It is the skill of *übersetzen,* which means to "translate" and "ferry across a river, to take from one bank to the other."

Our capacity to reconstruct in the other culture in a meaningful way depends on our capacity to enter that culture from the inside, to have an emic understanding of its values, behaviors, and organisation, or at least to be guided by someone from the inside. If they indicate, one way or another, that "we don't do that here," we have three choices: we conform because we want to go along with the receiving culture and do not feel compromised by so doing; we conform, whether we feel compromised or not, because the other has the power to impose certain behavior; or we try to understand why for them it should be considered as normal. Then, by comparing that rationale with our own systems of normality, we can choose to accommodate wholly, adapt, or refuse wholly. We need to accept that our own culture, so familiar and so natural, is "strange" to others. They have an etic, and possible a very exact, appreciation of what the culture represents.

One key question concerns how far what we take for granted, what is deemed to be normal, is actually made explicit. If we assume implicitly that "everybody knows that" or "obviously the best thing to do is . . .", it is highly probable that such an assumption fails to acknowledge the degree of difference explicit in an international exchange. We can almost plot an arc of imagination to reveal the contours of our practise (Figure 1.3). The more rules, procedures, norms, and values are *explicitly* recognised by the group, the more there will be an acceptance of the inherent differences within the group. Or, conversely, the degree of recognition of differences in the group will be directly related to the degree to which cultural/national assumptions are expressed and clarified.

A group that does not recognise cultural/national boundaries risks being oppressive. The claim that we are all the same and that everyone is equal is as dangerous as that which mistakes difference for incompatibility. Wisdom exists in the view that, for personal relationships as well as for group relationships, we need to find enough things that we have in common in order to be able to talk to one an-

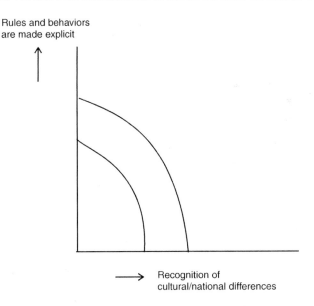

FIGURE 1.3. International Relationship Arc

other. But, equally, we need to find enough differences so that we will each have something to say. The word, says Bakhtin, is one-half of the other; it takes two to dialogue, just as it takes two cultures/nations to create a cross-cultural frontier. We can stay behind it, or we can cross over it, but first we have to know it is there. "Being foreign" is a view from here, looking over there, but from over there, we also seem foreign. If, in this symposium and later in our day-to-day practise, we can begin to explore what our own "foreignness" is about, how we behave ourselves, what we take for truth and common sense, we will at least begin to build our half of the bridge.

Let us start with the foundations. Let us look at our own procedures for organising power and individuality in groups, for being gender aware, and for responding to uncertainty and challenge. Crossing cultural and national boundaries may be like seeking the Promised Land, but, as Alinsky used to say, "There are those who say 'I will believe it when I see it.' That is not true. They will only see it when they believe it."

NOTES

1. Berque, A. (1996). *Etre humains sur la terre: Principes d'éthique de l'écumène*. Paris: Gallimard.

2. For the idea of overdetermination, (surdétermination, Uberdeterminierung), see Althusser, L. (1969). *For Marx*. London: Allen Lane.

3. A more detailed analysis is contained in Taylor, P. (1994). The linguistic and cultural barriers to cross-national groupwork. *Groupwork*, 7(1), 7-22.

4. Bollinger, D. and Hofstede, G. (1987). *Les différences culturelles dans le management*. Paris: Edition d'Organisation.

5. Tuckman, B. (1965). Development sequence in small groups. *Psychological Bulletin*, 63(6), 384-399. Some practitioners add a fifth stage to the "Forming–Storming–Norming–Performing," that of "Mourning" or "Ending." Others, following Woodcock, for example (Woodcock, M. [1981]. *Organisation Development Through Teambuilding*. London: Gower), focus more on the early stages of group life: "ritual sniffing, infighting, experimentation, effectiveness, and maturity."

6. The matrix is in fact a "diabolic" square, a mathematician's delight because the square remains diabolic even if a row is moved from top to bottom or if a column is moved from one side to the other. Any four adjacent cells on the field, up and down, left and right, or diagonally, will give the same result.

7. For a more detailed analysis, see the very useful discussion in Scollon, R. and Wong Scollon, S. (1995). *Intercultural Communication*. Oxford, UK: Blackwell, pp. 33-49.

8. Taylor. The linguistic and cultural barriers, p. 9.

9. See Tajfel, H. and Turner, J. (1979). An integrative theory of intergroup conflict. In Austin, W.G. and Worchel, S. (Eds.), *The Social Psychology of Intergroup Relations*. Pacific Grove, CA: Brooks/Cole; Headland, T., Pike, K., and Harris, M. (Eds.) (1990). *Emics and Etics: The Insider/Outsider Debate*. Newbury Park, CA: Sage; and Atmanspacher, H. and Dalenoort, G. (1994). *Inside versus Outside*. Berlin: Springer-Verlag.

10. Wright Mills, C. (1983). *L'imagination sociologique*. Paris: Maspero, p. 10.

11. Taylor, P. and Pineau, G. (1995). Pour une pédagogie de l'interculturel. In Leray, C. and Lorand, E. (Eds.), *Dynamique interculturelle et autoformation*. Paris: l'Harmattan.

Chapter 2

Crossing Boundaries:
Group Work with Persons with AIDS
in Early Recovery from Substance Abuse

Lawrence Shulman

Complex problems often require complex solutions. The time is past when a single profession or practice model can provide the help needed by many of our clients. Social work group workers have long recognized that the whole is more than the sum of its parts and that a unique synergy takes place when more than one person is involved in the helping process. For this reason, the theme of this year's symposium is most appropriate as we explore the many ways in which we and our clients can cross boundaries in order to increase the effectiveness of our practice.

In this chapter, I would like to provide an example that illustrates the crossing of a number of boundaries. For the past two years I have been a Faculty Fellow at the Boston University School of Social Work, participating with a number of my colleagues in a faculty development program sponsored by CSAP, the federal government's Center for Substance Abuse Prevention. In the second year of this project, each faculty fellow developed an individualized "fieldwork" experience. I chose to work with a multiservice agency, AIDS Action in Boston, coleading a group of clients with AIDS who were also in the early stage of substance abuse recovery.

John, my coleader, is a full-time, trained substance abuse counselor with the agency and is not a social worker. As an academic, I am primarily involved in teaching and research. John is in recovery; I am not. He is experienced in twelve-step programs such as Alcoholics Anonymous and Narcotics Anonymous and employs the organization's philosophy and recovery strategies. I have helped to develop a social work, mutual aid support group model, an approach that was relatively new to my coleader. He is African American and I am white and Jewish. Thus, as we worked together, we were crossing boundaries of professional disciplines, town and gown, practice orientation, life experience, race and ethnicity. Each of these differences would create obstacles we needed to deal with and provide the impetus for our own professional and personal growth. Working together across these boundaries profoundly affected our practice and thus the impact on our group members.

The five members of the client group had areas of common ground as well as boundaries they needed to bridge. What they all had in common was that they were persons with AIDS, they were in early recovery from prolonged polysubstance abuse (alcohol, cocaine, heroin, etc.), they had all been homeless and living on the streets, and most had been involved in either prostitution or crime to support their habits, and as emerged during the course of the group, they had all experienced some form of childhood victimization. What also emerged during the group was that they all had demonstrated significant resilience in the face of life experiences that I, as an outsider, could only begin to grasp.

Their differences created their own version of boundaries that they needed to cross as well. For example, early recovery for these clients ranged from one day clean and sober (one member insisted he could handle a drink once in a while) to the beginning of the second year, what one member described as "the year of the feelings." This was the year she indicated that you start to face all of the feelings you have used addictive substances to avoid. Using a stage change model described by Prochaska and DiClemente (1986), their readiness to deal with their addictions ranged from the "contemplative stage," considering making changes in their addictive behavior, to the "action stage," taking significant steps to deal with their addiction. The group met in a special residence that provided independent living with support for persons with AIDS. Three of the five members lived in the residence.

Group composition differences created boundaries as well. Members included Kerry, a twenty-eight-year-old white gay male; Tania, a forty-four-year-old white transgendered woman; Theresa, a twenty-six-year-old white heterosexual woman; Jake, a forty-two-year-old African-American male; and Gerry, a thirty-three-year-old African-

American male who had to leave the group at one point for two weeks to enter a residential detox program.

Differences also existed in relation to their struggle with the "virus," as they referred to AIDS. Jake and Gerry were included as subjects in a drug-testing protocol and were receiving the new triple-drug AIDS therapy. They had evidenced significant drops in their viral loads (the amount of the HIV virus in their system) and significant increases in their T-cell counts, which measures the strength of the antibodies that would fight the opportunistic infections which eventually could kill them. For these two members, the issues were living with AIDS and the deeply poignant question raised at one session, "Is it possible? Am I cured of the virus?"

Theresa, on the other hand, was waiting for her viral load and T-cell count to reach the levels required to enter the drug test subject group. She was battling weight loss and other physical symptoms but was hopeful that the therapy would eventually reverse her decline. Kerry was refusing to take the new drug therapy even though one look at his physical condition suggested that he should qualify for inclusion. Tania, our transgendered member, after years of drugging and the use of hormones, had too many physiological problems to be given the new treatment. For Tania, it was, in her words, "waiting to die" and trying to stay drug free so that she could take some control over the part of her life that remained.

For the group members, the boundaries to be crossed included gender, age, race, sexual orientation, commitment to and stage of recovery, degree of illness, living arrangements, individual prognosis, and their commitment to life. As will be illustrated later in the process recording excerpts, their differences created obstacles to overcome as well as the energy for change.

LITERATURE REVIEW

A little over ten years ago, Googins (1984) identified a syndrome that he described as the "Avoidance of the Alcoholic Client." He argued that while "problem drinkers" made up 12 percent of the population (21 percent of men and 5 percent of women, p. 161), social workers and their organizations tended to avoid offering service to this population, or even recognizing the problem in their clients when masked by other issues. Although this "avoidance" has been somewhat abated by programs such as the one that sponsored the CSAP faculty development program, his original assessment appears still to hold true.

In attempting to understand this reluctance to deal with this specific social problem, Googins identifies a number of "myths" surrounding alcoholism. For example, informational myths leave many people unable to appreciate that alcohol is a drug with properties and characteristics common to all drugs. Googins also identified "attitudinal myths" that lead to a moralizing approach which labels alcoholics as "morally inferior." Other attitudes, according to Googins (1984), lead to alcoholics being seen as "undesirable, untreatable and unmotivated" (p. 163).

Organizations that have labored long and hard to fill the treatment gap in the substance abuse field have been the self-help groups, such as Alcoholics Anonymous (AA), Narcotics Anonymous (NA), and a number of groups focusing on family members and friends of addicted persons, such as Al-Anon. Although these groups may differ in some ways, common themes emerge: a focus on achieving and maintaining sobriety and helping others to do so as well, the use of structure to help bind anxiety, and the use of traditions and slogans to support recovery efforts. AA (1984), for example, describes its purpose as follows:

> Alcoholics Anonymous is a fellowship of men and women who share their experience, strength and hope with each other so that they may solve their common problem and help others recover from alcoholism. The only requirement for membership is a desire to stop drinking. . . . Our primary purpose is to stay sober and help others to achieve sobriety. (p. 2)

Many of these self-help groups use twelve-step models to identify the route needed to achieve and maintain sobriety. My coleader and members of the group would often refer to these steps as guidelines for behavior when faced with difficult choices in their relationships with others. For example, steps eight and nine provide a means for members to deal with their guilt over their past behaviors by having "Made a list of all persons we had harmed, and become willing to make amends to them all," and "Made direct amends to such people whenever possible, except when to do so would injure them or others." These principles were invoked one night when men in the group discussed their guilt over having had unprotected sex with women after they knew they were infected with AIDS.

AA follows an "abstinence" model which suggests that alcoholism is a disease. One of the many AA sayings that guides members in their recovery is "For an alcoholic, one drink is too many and a thousand are not enough" (p. 10). While there are disputes in the substance abuse field about the "disease model," a focus on abstinence, the emphasis on spirituality, and other issues in twelve-step programs, this structured recovery program and philosophy has worked for many and was crucial for three of our group members who attended AA and NA meetings while also attending our group. In addition, when the recovery of any member appeared to be threatened, group members and my coleader drew upon their twelve-step experience to protect the recovery.

Matano and Yalom (1991) address the issue of crossing boundaries in their efforts to develop a synthesis of their "interactional" approach to group therapy and the methods employed by traditional chemical dependency groups. Although their interest is in a group therapy model in which the interpersonal interactions of the group members are used to develop insights and influence changes in interpersonal behaviors, a model somewhat different from the mutual aid support group described in this chapter, their principles for successful integration of approaches are relevant to this discussion. The authors suggest that

> an interactional approach can be effectively applied to alcoholics if the following guidelines are observed: (1) recovery is always accorded priority, (2) the patient accepts identification as an alcoholic, (3) anxiety is carefully modulated, (4) the proper distinction is made between what the alcoholic is and is not responsible for, (5) the therapist is thoroughly familiar with Alcoholics Anonymous language, steps, and traditions. It is important that therapists not permit misperceptions of AA to be used as therapy resistance and that they be able to harness the wisdom of AA for psychotherapeutic ends. (p. 269)

Many of the principles derived from Matano and Yalom's experience in group therapy apply to the effort described in this chapter and will be highlighted in the presentation.

Finally, Hardesty and Greif (1994) described the common themes in groups for female IV drug users who were HIV positive. They drew upon their work with a mandatory women's group in a methadone maintenance clinic. They note:

> Substance abuse spanned a number of generations. Members discussed with the group their long histories of physical abuse and neglect at the hands of family members, friends, and strangers, which left an indelible impression of worthlessness that the women carry into their current relationships with their parents, friends, lovers and children. Because of their belief in their own worthlessness, they fiercely guard secrets of shame and inadequacy. (p. 290)

The authors point out the unique advantages of a women's group in creating a safe environment for disclosure of family of origin issues.

Both women in the group described in the present chapter clearly expressed their struggles with feelings of self-worth that resulted in a vicious cycle of behaviors which maintained and often deepened their internalized negative views. When the dual stigmas of substance abuse and HIV are added, it is easy to understand their self-destructive behaviors and to marvel at their capacity for resilience.

THE WORK

In this section, I share illustrations from my process recordings of the group. They were dictated from my notes immediately following each session. I highlight the impact of boundary crossing for both the coleaders and the members associated with each excerpt.

The Formation Stage: Developing a Common Group Purpose

I have discussed elsewhere (Shulman, 1999) the tasks of the group leader and group members in the beginning phase. I have suggested that members bring a series of questions to a first session: Who are these leaders and what kind of people will they be? What is the purpose of this group and do I feel any connection to my sense of urgency and my current needs? Who are these other group members and what kind of people will they be? Do I share anything in common with them? I have described the worker's tasks in the first session as clarifying the group's purpose and the role of the worker, addressing authority theme concerns such as confidentiality, inviting feedback from the members as they attempt to find connections to the group's purpose and the other members, and developing a positive and supportive culture for work. I illustrate these dynamics and skills in the sections that follow.

Our first efforts at contracting were directed at clarifying the purpose of the group and identifying the potential connections each member had with the group service and with one another. The purpose was explained to members in the recruitment interviews and in the first session as follows:

> There are groups for persons with AIDS and there are groups for people in early recovery from substance abuse. This is a support group for persons who are dealing with both. The focus will be on how your recovery issues and your AIDS issues affect each other. We know a number of you attend AA or NA, as well as other groups to support your recovery, and we encourage you to continue to attend these groups if you find them helpful. The difference in this group is that you will be able to discuss your AIDS issues as well, something you may not feel confortable doing in your other groups. We think that as you help one another in this group, you will be helping yourselves.

For my coleader, this notion of mutual aid and members helping one another deal with specific life problems, emotions, and cognitions that affected their lives was a new and interesting concept. His experience had been mostly in the twelve-step model in which, for example, one person presents his or her drinking and/or drugging experiences, often called the "drunkalogue," and speakers from the group share their collective wisdom of the stages of recovery and strategies for maintaining recovery. Person-to-person help might be provided by an individual substance abuse counselor or a twelve-step sponsor; however, "cross-talk" was specifically discouraged. Help with individual problem solving is not considered appropriate in the group meeting. The support of the group was evidenced in more general ways, for example, the warm welcome expressed by the group in chorus in response to a new member introducing himself or herself. However, discussion of an individual's problems in living and problem solving is not encouraged in twelve-step groups.

As our group developed it became clear that issues of early trauma also would emerge in the discussion. For example, Tania, our transgendered female member, described how when she discovered she was really a woman, at age seventeen, her working-class family reacted violently to her revelation. At first, her parents had her admitted to a psychiatric hospital where electric shock therapy was used to try to "straighten her out." (This was twenty years ago and I would like to think it would not happen today . . . but who knows.) In another incident, her older brother took a gun and held it to her head, threatening to kill her if she did not move away and stop "shaming the family." For Tania, as with all of the members, family issues and unresolved trauma-related experiences have played a significant part in their addictions and in their lives.

My interventions, based upon my experience leading support groups, helped my coleader see how the exploration of feelings and cognitions that affected current day-to-day coping could help members take more control over their lives and take responsibility for their part in their intimate relationships. This empowerment over their lives helped them to keep control of their recovery and not, as one member put it, "Hand my recovery over to someone else."

On the other hand, the personal and professional experiences of my substance abuse counselor coleader led us to encourage our members to be cautious in their disclosures in order to ensure that they were able to modulate their anxiety so as not to threaten their own recovery or the recovery of other members who might be at a different stage in the process. Coleading with an experienced substance abuse counselor taught me the importance of always keeping the recovery issues front and center and to tread gently, where I might have pushed harder, in areas our clients might not be ready to handle.

To return to our first group session, after some discussion of confidentiality issues, the group members began to share some of their life issues, which represented their feedback to our opening statement and our offer to work. Since we had purposely started the group just before the Thanksgiving holiday, it was not surprising that coping with holidays, families, loneliness, and sobriety were early issues. In these first excerpts you will note that I continually reach for the feelings associated with the member's comments, and John, my coleader, clarifies issues related to recovery. Our collaboration began with each of us influencing the work of the group and each other. The excerpt continues with what I have called problem swapping (Shulman, 1999), group members sharing their responses to our offer.

Jake jumped in and said he wanted to tell a story about what had happened over the weekend. He had gone home to visit his family in another town in the state. He said, "I couldn't stay. They started to make me crazy right away. Everyone there was drinking and drugging, and I knew, if I stayed, they would pull me in, and I can't let them pull me in. I have to fight that. I know I can't control this. If I take one drink or use drugs once, I'm going to be back to going into the bar at eight in the morning and staying right through until two a.m. drinking myself to death."

I said that it sounded like, in addition to giving up the drinking and drugging, he was also having to give up his family. He agreed. Kerry said that he had been in a bar in the last week and had two drinks. He said, "I can handle that. Just because I have two drinks doesn't mean I am going to go back to where I was a year ago. I know you people are going to say I am in denial, but it's not true. I know I can handle this." John, my coleader, said that we had to understand that recovery was different for each person and that we had to make room in the group for people to feel safe and not defensive as they described their own ways of handling their recovery. I nodded in agreement. The rest of the group did as well.

Theresa jumped in at that point and said that she was not living at this residence. She was living in a single-room-occupancy building two blocks away. She said that most of the people in that building were active users and, for her, it was a fight every day to make sure that she didn't get pulled in. She said that she knew that she didn't want to go back to all the drinking and drugging she had been doing. She told us that she had gotten out of the penitentiary after a five-year sentence, and that in the penitentiary she had dried out and learned not to use. She said that she didn't want to go back to when she hated herself and she would spend her time on street corners sucking old men's dicks in order to get enough money for a shot of crack. Tania agreed, and said that when she thought of some of the things she did for the ten-year period that she was drinking and drugging all the time, she couldn't believe she actually let herself do those things. Theresa said, "I still have to deal with the housing, even though I am not in this residence, but I know the real question is how we deal with ourselves. For me, religion has been the answer."

THE AUTHORITY THEME

In any first session, early issues for the group revolve around their relation to the group leaders, what I have referred to as the authority theme (Shulman, 1999), the ongoing struggle of group members to

come to grips with the group leaders as demanding and yet supportive symbols of authority. In this first session, the authority theme
emerged as group members needed to deal with me, the stranger, and
the question of whether or not I had "walked the walk," been a substance abuser, and "talked the talk," participated in a twelve-step
group. Some members already knew that my coleader, who served as
their individual substance abuse counselor, was in recovery, but my
status was unknown. The question emerged, as it often does, in an indirect way.

Tania went on about all the holiday parties that were going on, and how
difficult it was for her to party. She said, "I don't know how to party without
first drinking and drugging. As I looked at the people at this party I attended
last week, through clean and sober eyes, I said, 'My God, was this me? Was
this the way I lived my life?' I left the party when they started passing around
the cocaine, because if I had stayed, I might have given in." (Tania was only
one month into her recovery and still obviously very shaky.) "I know you all
know what I'm talking about, since you're in recovery as well, although I don't
know about them [pointing toward us]."

I decided to use this as an opportunity to address the authority theme and
to review the limits of confidentiality. I pointed out that Tania had mentioned a
couple of times her concern about confidentiality, and also had raised the
question indirectly about whether we were in recovery. I said that I would
have to speak for myself.

"I'm not in recovery so I am an outsider." I went on to say that I thought the
issue of trust with myself and John was a major one for them today, and they
were worried about whether an "outsider" like myself could understand and
were concerned about what we might share outside of the group. I pointed
out that for three of them, they were concerned that we might divulge information that would affect their ability to continue in a clean and sober residence. They agreed that they wanted to hold onto their apartments, which
were the best of this type available to people with AIDS in the city.

I told them that I was a social worker and that I taught social work at the
university. I told them I had asked John and AIDS Action if it were possible for
me to colead this group because I thought it was important that as a teacher
I continued to work directly with people. Tania exploded and said, "I thought
you were a narc." I laughed and said, "A narc? You mean I look like a narcotics detective?" She continued, "I thought you were just going to sit there,
take notes and, right after this session, you were going to march me off to the
police station and that I'd be arrested." I laughed again and said, "Look [hold-
ing my sweater up], no wire and no badge." They all laughed. I said, "I'm not a
narc, but it's going to take a while for you to really believe and trust that we
will keep what you raise here confidential, except for those conditions we
mentioned earlier . . . if you are involved in an illegal activity in the house,
such as selling dope, or if you are a danger to yourself or to others. I'm hoping we can earn your trust." Their heads were nodding in agreement.

My coleader John asked the members of the group if they were ready to sign an agreement we had discussed about such issues as attendance and confidentiality. They said they were ready, and I said, "Maybe we should sign as well."

The authority theme would emerge often in the group in later sessions in many different ways. Once members felt safer with me, and when I responded directly to indirect cues from group members, we would explore its implications for our differences in gender, race, sexual orientation, class, and status. The authority theme remained a powerful source of energy for our work right until the last session I attended, as we discussed our ending and what the group had meant to me and to the members.

THE INTIMACY THEME:
HELPING YOURSELF BY HELPING OTHERS

In addition to their relationship to the leader, group members must also work on their relationship to one another, what I have described elsewhere (Shulman, 1999) as the intimacy theme. Bennis and Sheppard (1956) refer to the conflict to decide the level of intimacy members are willing to risk with the group's ambivalence expressed by members who are "counterpersonal," resisting intimacy, and those who are "overpersonal," wanting more intimacy. In the excerpts that follow, Tania at first expresses the counterpersonal force while Theresa attempts to lead the group into a deeper level of intimacy.

The struggle was evident in the group members' willingness to address their AIDS. Although many powerful themes emerged in the first few meetings, the group members seemed to avoid discussion of AIDS. When it did emerge, it was mentioned briefly, with members quickly changing the subject. In Bion's (1961) terms, the unsophisticated group would turn to "fight" or "flight" as a way of avoiding the underlying pain. In addition, a pattern developed of group members presenting problems while the others listened in a generally supportive manner. The idea of the group staying with a particular member's concern and offering specific help was foreign to them. Although members acknowledged and empathized with expressed concerns and experiences, they often quickly shared their own versions of the issue. They appeared to use a model they were comfortable with from their twelve-step experiences. During these sessions my coleader focused on maintenance of recovery issues, while I continued to reach, sometimes successfully, often unsuccessfully, for the mutual aid potential.

One member, Jake, started bringing in handouts that he shared with members at the end of each meeting. These were used in twelve-step groups he attended and provided recovery advice and philosophy. It was not until the fifth session that he finally told me, in a gentle manner, that he was bringing the handouts to help me out since I "obviously didn't know how to lead a recovery group." I thanked him and told him I could use all the help I could get.

An important turning point in the group came in this fifth session. My coleader and I had agreed at our last postgroup meeting to confront the group with the avoidance of AIDS discussion and to recontract on the purpose and structure of the group. By attending the group and accepting us as leaders, and accepting one another, our group members had made what I call the "first decision." We would now be asking them to make the "second decision"; in this one, they needed to make the transition from the beginning phase to the work phase. The work phase would be characterized by a deepening of the discussion and a clearer sense of mutual aid. Unfortunately, my coleader was ill the night of the next meeting. We spoke by phone and he agreed I should proceed with our strategy. My record of the session follows.

Session Five

Kerry, Jake, and Tania were in the lobby when I arrived. Tania was angry because John (my coleader) was not going to be there that evening. She said she had business with him. I pointed out that he would be at the meeting the next week and I would be glad to pass along her concerns. She said, "I don't think I'm coming to the meeting." She was in a bathrobe and looked terrible physically. She said she wasn't feeling well but said she would come for just the beginning. I spoke to Kerry, who was sulking as well, saying he could only come for the first half hour. I discussed his holidays with him for a few minutes and, at one point, he complained about the group as being just "bitching sessions," and then he said, "Some people [and he secretively pointed toward Tania] talk too much." I told him I understood what he was raising and that I would be dealing with it today. Jake was talking to another resident during this time. He joined us when we went upstairs.

Theresa arrived. Tania said, "Maybe we should fill the people who weren't here in on what happened last week." Then she turned to me and said, "But I'm doing your job, aren't I?" I encouraged her to continue. She filled in John and Theresa about the discussion they had concerning the residence and some of their issues about the group. I said I wanted to raise a question right at the beginning. I had spoken to John and we felt it was important to find out whether or not there was a real commitment to the group. I knew that some members had only come because they believed they had to come or risk losing their housing. (Tania and Kerry had recently relapsed and were mandated to enter some form of treatment, this group being one option.) Tania said, "I suppose it helps to sit around and bitch each week. I guess that makes me feel a little bit better."

I told her that was not the purpose of the group, and that I wanted to restate the purpose to see whether or not we had some agreement on it. I pointed out, once again, that it was a group for people who were dealing with both the virus and early recovery, and how one affected the other. Tania said she didn't think that was the group's purpose. Theresa said, yes, that was exactly what she understood it to be, a place where she could deal with the impact of her having the virus.

I went on to tell them that, unless this group could become a place where they could be helpful to one another, where they could make connections, and be supportive to one another, it would not succeed. I told them that the purpose of the group was to help them figure out how to deal with some of the difficult issues in their lives they were raising each week, not just to complain about them. I said I knew it was hard to set aside some of your own concerns and invest yourself in someone else's issues, but that's what the group was about. I said I thought all of them had problems in their lives in trying to get close and make connections to people, and that this group was a place for them to relearn how to do that. I went on to say that the group would not be valuable unless they could learn to really care for one another. I pointed out that most of them had described experiences where they were exploited by people or they exploited people, and that trust in others was difficult. I said it seemed that their most serious connection in recent years was the one they had with drugs and booze, and that making connections was what the group was all about.

Theresa enthusiastically said that that's why she wants help from the group, that's what she needs help with. She said she wanted to talk about her boyfriend and the impact of her HIV on the relationship. As she was talking, Tania interrupted her and started to complete her sentences.

I decided it was time to draw on the positive relationship I felt I had developed over the first four meetings and stopped the group and pointed this out. I tried to make what I call an "empathic demand for work." While confronting Tania, I simultaneously acknowledged what I believed to be her underlying feelings.

I said, "Tania, you know, you haven't let Theresa finish a sentence. I could be wrong, but I think you get very anxious about these discussions and that talking is a way of dealing with it." She said, "Oh, did I?" and made as if to zipper her mouth and put her hand over it. I told her I would help her because I thought she had a lot to give, but I thought other people needed the chance to get involved as well. Tania accepted this and, for the rest of the evening, actively tried to catch herself when she was jumping in or cutting people off.

Theresa started to talk about her concerns. She said she was eighteen months clean and sober, and so she was in the middle of the second year, which was a "feelings year." She went on to describe that this was the period when she and, she thought, everyone in recovery started to face all those feelings they had been running from. She said it was a complex and difficult time, and that it was hard to sort things out. She went on to say that her boyfriend had trouble sharing his feelings with her. When she wanted to talk to her boyfriend about issues, like her AIDS, he pulled back and told her it was too painful. As a result, she would back off. She knows he's experienced a lot of losses, including the death of his wife from illness fairly recently, and she realizes he is still early in recovery, but she has things she wants to talk to him about. She has a closeness she wants to achieve. She has some commitments she wants from him and she is afraid that he can't make commitments at this point. He's holding back. I asked the others in the group if they had any advice for Theresa on this issue.

Theresa had spoken with great emotion and I was determined not to do "casework in the group" and instead to wait for members to respond. Kerry, who usually sits quietly at the meetings, and who indicated that he was going to leave as soon as he could, jumped right in. (This was after I once again slowed Tania down and told her I would direct traffic and help her keep herself under control.)

Kerry said he thought that her boyfriend was having trouble dealing with his losses and it wasn't easy. He described a very close relationship with his partner, Billy, that ended two years ago, when his partner died of AIDS on Christmas Day. He said he still didn't think he'd come to grips with all the feelings that he had and the loss that he'd experienced. I said that must make each Christmas even more difficult for him, and he agreed. He went on to talk about how he had been raised by an extremely physically abusive mother and that his grandmother was the only person who provided him with any support and love. He said he didn't think he had gotten over her dying either. He told Theresa that she had to realize that the process takes a long time and that it might not be easy for her boyfriend to discuss it with her, because he knew it wasn't easy for him to discuss his loss with other people.

As Kerry talked, I saw a sensitive and caring side of him that he keeps covered up with his abrasive, grandiose, angry front, with his consistently telling us he doesn't need anybody and, if they don't care about him, "the hell with them."

Theresa acknowledged his comments and thanked Kerry for sharing that with her, as did the other members of the group. Tania came in at that point and reinforced what Kerry had been saying. Jake was shaking his head as if he understood that difficulty as well.

Whenever a group member raises a general problem there is usually a specific, recent example that is creating a sense of urgency. I attempted to help Theresa elaborate on her "first offering" by using a skill I call "reaching from the general to the specific" (Shulman, 1999).

I asked Theresa if anything had happened recently to make her feel so strongly about this issue. Theresa described an incident that led to a major fight with her boyfriend. They were in a car together and she was in the backseat. There was another woman in the front seat whom she experienced as coming on to her boyfriend. The woman was asking him when they could get together and how much she'd like to "bump and grind" with him on the dance floor. Every time Theresa described this woman's comments, she did an imitation of her, making it sound flirtatious and seductive. Theresa went on with a great deal of anger, saying that her boyfriend didn't even acknowledge that she was in the backseat and that she was his woman. Therefore, this woman, a friend of his, was going on right in front of her, which she felt was "disrespecting" her. She thought her boyfriend was "disrespecting" her by not stopping the woman and not being aware of her feelings.

I asked if she had talked to her boyfriend about this, and she said she had, but he had just told her that she was "insecure." Theresa said, "Look, I don't know how to deal with this. I try to use a prayer I know from the twelve-step program. Maybe I can pray he can change. But I don't think he's going to change because, even though he is in a twelve-step program, I don't think he's really committed to it. I think he can talk the talk, but he doesn't walk the walk. He's got all the words, but he doesn't practice any of it. I'm not sure he's going to change at all."

Theresa continued, "I realize for both of us this is our first recovery relationship, and I know I have to be patient because he's not where I am in recovery, but still it's very hard to sit in the car and have him disrespect me in that way." She said that she was absolutely furious at this woman and that maybe she ought to go have a talk with the lady. She had a great deal of anger as she described the fact that she was just recently released from the penitentiary, and there she learned how to fight (pointing to her two missing lower teeth). She said, "I can ask this lady nicely first, but if I don't get anywhere, then it's my boot up her ass."

As Theresa's anger grew I was aware of her pattern, one mirrored by most group members, of using what Bion (1961) described as "fight or flight" to deal with pain. Substance abuse itself is a form of flight and violence is a form of fight. These are maladaptive approaches to coping with the underlying feelings and cognitions and have proved to be devastating to these group members. Most have been employing these techniques to cope with the deep pain and emotional damage of persistent exploitation and oppression related to gender, sexual orientation, race, and class. My goal was to help the members to become aware of their maladaptive defensive maneuvers. I made use of the idea from twelve-step programs of the primacy of maintaining control over your recovery.

I asked Theresa if that would solve the problem, since it might get rid of this woman, but if she doesn't resolve the issues with her boyfriend, wouldn't there just be another one? She agreed and seemed a bit deflated. I said that it seemed to me she had to talk to her boyfriend. Also, her anger was so strong that if she did take physical action against this other woman, she might be risking her own recovery and even her freedom, and the last thing she wanted to do was to end up back in prison on an assault charge. She nodded her head and said, "I know it would mean I'd be losing control of my recovery and giving it to someone else, but I don't know if I could talk to him or if he'll listen to me without just putting me off."

Tania then spoke with great feeling about what an important and wonderful person that Theresa was, and that she deserved respect and that, if she respected herself, which Tania thought she did, then she should stand up for herself and not let this guy get away with this. She had to tell him directly that she wanted him to make a commitment to her, to recognize her as his woman. Also, if there were these kinds of issues, she had to deal with them out in the open and couldn't let them just fester where she would get angrier and angrier. She said, "If you continue to get this angry, you're just going to hurt yourself, you're going to get sick, and eventually you're going to threaten your recovery." Theresa agreed that this was going to be a problem for her.

Although Theresa had presented a very real and painful problem, she still had not focused on her AIDS, even though she had said at the start of the session that she wanted to address it. I was conscious of this as I tried to explore why she had accepted the current situation with her boyfriend. I was making what Schwartz (1961) described as a "demand for work" and what I have called a facilitative confrontation (Shulman, 1999). It was a gentle demand in which I asked Theresa to examine her reasons for not pursuing the issues.

I asked Theresa why she let her boyfriend back off when she asked him to talk about his losses and her AIDS. She said, "Well, he told me it was hard to talk about." I responded, "Well, you could have asked him what made it hard. Why do you give up when he resists conversations with you?" There was a long silence and then Theresa's face softened and she said, "I guess I really don't want to hear." Everyone in the room nodded their heads in agreement. I said, "Good for you, Theresa. Now you're taking some responsibility. What are you afraid you're going to hear?" She went on and said, "I'm afraid I'm going to be rejected."

Jake jumped in at that point, with a lot of emotion, and said, "That's the problem when you've got the virus. People reject you." He went on and talked about his own family and how he'd gotten in trouble with the law over a fight and he was in court and nobody knew him in that court. He said he was about to get released without having to do jail time because of the fight. He said, "My own mother was in the court and she hurt me deeply—she really pained me—when she stood up and told the judge that I was HIV positive. Well, that changed everything. These people got real angry at me, and they didn't want a guy getting into fights who was HIV positive, who had the AIDS bug, and they said, 'Go to jail' . . . I couldn't believe the rejection I felt from my mother. I tried to explain it to her later, and she didn't understand that I didn't want her telling people I was HIV positive, not in those circumstances." He then turned to Theresa and said, "So, I can understand why you're afraid of that rejection. . . . I think we're all afraid of what people will do once they know we've got the virus." (At a later meeting Jake told us the fight was with a drug dealer who had murdered his sister and had successfully avoided arrest.)

Tania had been very quiet, although I could tell she wanted to speak. At one point, I said, "I think Tania wants to get in here, and she's been well-behaved this session, we have to give her a chance." She smiled and jumped in, telling Theresa how much she admired her, and how much strength she had, and that she hoped that she could handle her own recovery in the way that Theresa was handling hers. She told Theresa that she just deserved a lot more.

Theresa asked Tania whether she thought she was an attractive person. There was a silence and Tania said, "I think you're a beautiful young woman and you could have any man you want." Theresa went on at some length about how men come on to her and, if she wanted to, she could "bump and grind" with them as well, but she didn't want that. She wanted one relationship. She wanted a serious relationship. She said she was getting older now and she wanted a commitment from someone and this was just not enough, and that was what the issue was all about.

Jake, our often quiet yet very thoughtful member, had changed the norm and broken the taboo by raising the fear of rejection associated with AIDS. Theresa's question to Tania about her looks was an indirect way of getting at the issue of fear of rejection. I tried to facilitate her expression by articulating her feelings.

I said to Theresa, "Is the question really that you're afraid that he might not stay with you, that, if you actually confront him on this issue of the other woman, he might leave you?" She agreed that it was her concern. At this point, I wondered if it might help Theresa to figure out what she might say to her boyfriend. Theresa said that would be helpful because she didn't know when and how to say it. Then she laughed and said, "Maybe I should say it in bed." Tania said, "Oh no. Don't say it before sex and don't say it after sex." And I added, "And don't say it during sex." Everyone laughed and Tania did a hilarious imitation of having a conversation with Theresa's boyfriend, while pumping up and down, as if she were in bed having sex with him.

After the laughter died down Tania said, "You have to find a quiet time, not a time when you're in the middle of a fight, and you have to just put out your feelings." I asked Tania if she could show Theresa how she could do that. She started to speak as if she were talking to Theresa's boyfriend. I role-played the boyfriend, and said, "Oh, but Theresa you're just insecure, aren't you?" Tania did a very good job of not letting me put her off and, instead, put the issue right where it was, whether or not Theresa's boyfriend was prepared to make a commitment or if he was too insecure.

Theresa listened carefully and then said, "I know I have to talk to him, but, you know, he told me that he's not sure he wants to be tied down, that he likes to have his freedom." Jake nodded his head and said, "Yeah, that's the problem. They want their freedom and they don't want to make a commitment, and you're afraid, if you push him, he'll leave you because you've got the virus." Theresa said she realized she had to sit down and talk to him because it couldn't keep up the same way. She would just get too angry and do something crazy and screw up her recovery. She felt she had to find another way to get through to him and talk to him. Otherwise, this thing was just going to continue and it was going to tear her up inside.

The session was approaching the ending phase and I wanted to bring the maintenance of recovery issue front and center. This normally would have been a focus of John, my missing coleader. In Tania's moving response to Theresa, we can see the dynamic of "resonance," as described by Fidele (1994) in her discussion of women's groups and "relational theory," as a resounding or echoing and a capacity for empathy.

I said, if she did confront him, it was going to be very rough for her, especially with the holiday, and I wondered whom she'd have for support if he said he didn't want to continue the relationship. She said she had her sponsor, and Tania said, "You also have me. You can call me anytime you want. . . . I didn't realize when I started this group there were people who have lived lives just like me, who had feelings just like me, who had struggles just like me. You—you're a woman—you've really helped me see that I'm just not the only one going through this. I'd do anything I could to help you."

Once again, Theresa asked Tania how she looked. She said, "You're a woman. I know, as a woman, you will be honest with me and just tell me what you think. Do you think I look okay?" Tania seemed confused and said, "Well, sure, you look wonderful." I said, "I wonder if Theresa is really asking, 'Am I pretty enough? Am I attractive enough? If my boyfriend leaves me, can I find someone else who could love me even though I have AIDS?' " She said, "That's it," and started to cry. She said, "I'm so afraid, if I lose him, I won't find anyone else. . . . I know I could have guys, and I know I could have sex, and I like the sex. I sure missed it during the time I was in prison, but can another guy love me?" A number of group members tried to reassure Theresa, with Tania summarizing by saying, "Theresa, it's not what you look like on the outside, it's what you're like on the inside, and you, honey, you've really got it where it counts."

As we were coming to an end, I asked them what they thought about the evening. I pointed out that some members had said they thought one hour was too long for a group, and yet we had gone an hour and a half. Theresa said everybody was really very helpful. Tania said, "You know, I didn't want to come, but it's turned out really to be okay." Jake said he really enjoyed tonight and he liked my leading the group. (This was the first session that Jake did not provide a twelve-step group handout.)

I credited Tania for her ability to contain herself, even though many times she felt like just jumping in and speaking. I told her I thought she had been very helpful and supportive in her comments. I also credited Kerry and Jake for sharing painful but very helpful parts of their lives. Finally, I acknowledged Theresa for taking a big risk and sharing her problem with us.

After the meeting ended, I spent a few minutes chatting with one of the staff members in the lobby. Tania came down to sit in the lobby area. She said, "This was a really good meeting," and held up her hand for me to give her a high-five slap. I left the session feeling we had experienced an important turning point in the group's development. I felt that the group members had made the "second decision" and were now in transition to the middle phase of work.

At the next meeting, attended by myself and my coleader, Theresa told me that she had relapsed during the week, a comment that initially shook my growing confidence in my work with this new population. I was concerned that I had not balanced work on strong emotional issues with attention to maintaining the member's recovery. My coleader John was very active in this session, bringing his experience dealing with threats to recovery as he supported Theresa in her struggle.

When I arrived, Theresa was waiting in the lobby, looking very distressed. She said she had almost used on the weekend (she has been eighteen months in recovery and has been an example to the other members). She said, instead of using drugs, she used a man. Since we were a few minutes early, I suggested we go up to the group room and she could tell me what had happened. Theresa sat in the high-backed armchair that Tania had sat in the week before and said, "I'm in Tania's chair."

She told me that she had broken up with her boyfriend, but she had done it in a way that she wasn't very proud of. He had been arrested over the weekend and his mother and daughter were in a car crash, so it was a tough weekend for him too. She had wanted to talk to him about what we had discussed at the last meeting (her anger over his "dissing" her in front of another woman), but he had been reluctant to do so. She said she was still very mad at him because of his disrespect for her, and that she realized now that her motives were really just to get even with him and to hurt him. When I asked her what she did, she said she had slept with another man, Jim, and that when she had called her boyfriend, she had left a message on his machine, telling him that they were breaking up and also telling him that she had slept with another man.

She said she knew this was not the way that we had suggested that she handle it—an understatement to say the least—that Tania had specifically said not to do it on the phone, to do it in person, but she'd just ignored the advice. She said she had been so distressed by this that the dope fiend in her took over, the illness took over, and she thought she had to use. Instead of using drugs, she had used a man. I acknowledged what a terrible weekend this was for her and asked her if she thought she could share this with the group because I knew they would be concerned about what had happened since last week. She said she would.

When I realized Theresa had not relapsed with drugs or alcohol I felt a wave of relief. I had felt an initial sense of guilt at the thought that at the first meeting I had handled alone I may have led a member to relapse. I've since realized I was not able to help or, for that matter, hurt that much. Theresa's recovery was in her own hands and she was going through an important stage in the process.

At 4:30, Jake and Tania arrived. Tania said to Theresa, "You're sitting in my chair." I told Tania I thought Theresa needed that chair this week. Tania immediately sat down next to her and reached out to her and said, "Was it a really bad week?" Theresa said that it was. My coleader John suggested that we start with thirty seconds of silence.

In the excerpts that follow, it is interesting to note that this threat to Theresa's recovery brought forth from the group and my coleader numerous comments from their own recovery experiences, making use of metaphors, philosophy, and sayings from their twelve-step programs. I had grown to respect these methods as powerful tools for providing structure at points of crisis.

Theresa told her story to the group members, her words full of strong emotions. Mostly, she said, she felt guilty for the way she had done it. She said, "My disturbed feelings, my addiction, my disease—they can tell me all kinds of lies, but in my heart, I know I did this to punish him, and I did it badly, and I'm feeling lousy about it. I'm feeling rotten. . . . I know I was angry at him and he disrespected me, but I cheated on him." She said she didn't feel her actions were justified. She continued to say she always felt that she had to be open in communication with other people because "you're as sick as your secrets," but, in this case, she thought her motives were just to hurt him. I said, "Because you felt he had hurt you." She agreed.

She said, "I'm really in love with him and now I think I have broken it up for good, and it's really upsetting, especially with Christmas coming." Tania, who had been sitting quietly, asked if she could speak. She turned to Theresa and said, "You were wrong to do it on the phone. It was a bad way to handle it, but you had a right to be angry and, remember, he started it." Theresa said she felt really guilty and out of control in the whole situation, and that all she could do now was pray and try to forgive herself. Tania said to Theresa, "You seem to be taking all the responsibility for this. Don't you think he had a part in it as well?" At that point, Theresa got angry again and said, "He did disrespect me. He didn't treat me right. He treated me like his 'ho' [whore], instead of his woman." Tania said, "I know it's rough and you didn't handle it well, but the point is, you're standing up for yourself. You're not letting him treat you like his ho. He wasn't ready to make a commitment to you. He kept ducking all the conversations when you tried to have one with him, so maybe it's better you brought it about now." John said, "You've got a lot of mixed emotions right here," and he described her ambivalence.

Theresa said that she had been faithful to her boyfriends even when she was using. She said, "Even when I was on the street tricking—I was with no man even while I was sleeping with a lot of men. . . . What I am upset about is that this weekend with Jim—I was a dope fiend with this man, I was using him, and that's just as bad as using drugs. . . . I don't know what to do. I am at a loss now. I know I started to put my boyfriend before my recovery. All I can do now is put it in the hands of God. I went to a meeting every day since I made that call and I called my sponsor, and she was helpful as well." Theresa continued, "I know you can't keep doing the same thing and looking for different results," and she said that this is what happens in all her relationships with men.

Tania, with a lot of emotion, told her that "using sex is not like using drugs." John said, to Tania, "You're taking it personally and it might be different for Theresa." Tania said, "She is not addicted to sex, so using a man during the weekend was not as dangerous as using drugs, because she is addicted to them." At this point, Theresa had gotten up to get a bagel and was standing in the room and laughed and said, "Who says I'm not addicted to sex?" And then she wiggled her hips and said, "I can be a little nymphomaniac if I want to."

I pointed out that Theresa has told us a number of things on one side of the ledger, she had stood up for herself and asked her boyfriend to treat her with respect and to not continue without commitment. On the other side, she had done it badly. On the good side, she hadn't used drugs, and she went to her resources—her sponsor, her meetings—so she took steps to stay in control. On the other side of the ledger, she used a guy, which she felt guilty and badly about. Theresa said, "I am upset and I am guilty, 'cause sex is like a drug for me."

As I have grown to understand, relapses are very much a part of the recovery process. The members and the group leaders attempted to help Theresa see that her choice of relapse was one which reduced the possible harm to her and her recovery. In the recovery process, the important thing is to learn from your relapse experiences.

Tania said, "Look, Theresa, if you did drugs, you wouldn't be here today." John asked how long she had been seeing this guy, Jim, and she said, "Not long at all." John said that it's not unusual to put a guy or a woman on the "layaway plan." "You come on a little, you let him know you're interested, and, when you need him later, you can cash him in."

I reminded everyone that Theresa had told us last week that one of her real fears of losing her boyfriend was that, because she had AIDS, she would not be able to find another man to love her. My coleader said, "You know, Theresa, what I am seeing in you is a lot of progress. You held on to your eighteen-month recovery. You didn't do the drugs. You were upset. You needed something, but you didn't collapse. You're taking responsibility for the motives about what you did and you're not trying to explain it away."

Theresa said she was just so angry at her boyfriend. I said, "I think you're also very angry at yourself." Tania said, "All I'm seeing right here is that you didn't use." John said, "You picked the lesser of two evils, but you picked the one that you could walk away from." Tania said, "Don't feel guilty about having slept with a guy. Men have been doing this for years. They don't worry about it. They get a lot of macho bullshit when they're sleeping with women, and it doesn't matter whether they care about them or not. Take my word for it, I've been both! I've been a guy and a woman, and I know that's all people care about—sex and money. When I was prostituting—and I'm not proud of that—for over twenty years I slept with judges, I slept with teachers, I slept with businessmen, I slept with politicians, and all they cared about was getting sex. If you have enough money, you can get sex."

John said, "Let's get back to what happened. Breaking up is really painful. It's one of the really difficult times when you're in recovery because you're going through all that pain and you can't use the drug to make it go away." Theresa said she also lost her sponsee, a fifteen-year-old that she was working with. She said the sponsee wanted to switch to another one—that she felt that Theresa was going through too much right now to help her. I said, "So, you've had a lot of rejection this week."

The meeting continued with Tania, Jake, and Kerry offering Theresa examples from their own life experiences where they had experienced similar rejections and how these had impacted them. They were reassuring her that her response was understandable and reminding her that she had chosen a less-damaging relapse. In Jake's story he described how he was used by a woman to get to his brother and how when he broke up with her he broke up with his brother as well. He went on to describe how he cut himself off to protect himself.

Jake said, "So, I've closed my door, shut off my phone, and I stay in my room and cut myself off because I know, if I try to get close, people are going to hurt me again, and then that's going to stop my recovery." I reminded everyone that Jake had said he had stayed home on Thanksgiving Day, cooked his own turkey, and just had his meal in his room. Jake said, "And I ate the whole thing." The group members all laughed with him.

Jake went on to say that going to school had given him a new direction. He told everyone in the group he had a great day today because the place he is training and working in picked him as employee of the month, and they have even said he's going to get the award as employee of the year. There was a great deal of pride in his face and voice as he described this. The rest of the group members all burst out in applause and said, "Way to go. Nice going, Jake." He went on to say, "I wear a suit when I go to work every day," and he pointed to the jacket he was wearing at the meeting, "because I want to dress right and feel good about myself. I've also wanted to stop taking on other people's nonsense."

He turned to Theresa and said, "For most men, it's tough not to think about women as just sexual objects and to treat them as if they had dignity." He said, when he didn't have any self-esteem himself, it was hard to treat women as equals, as persons you could really care about. I pointed out he was now getting a lot of his self-esteem from his work, and he agreed.

At this point, I said to the group it seemed to me that there was a struggle going on here. It was all or nothing. "You could have relationships with people and experience a lot of pain, a lot of rejection, especially with the AIDS virus, or do nothing, close your door, cut off your phone, don't have sex, just withdraw. The feeling I get is that you've rarely, if ever, had relationships with people who cared about you and didn't exploit you, and so, as far as you're concerned, there's no middle ground."

Tania turned to Jake on the couch and said, "You know, maybe if I could find a guy like you, Jake, a guy who could talk about his feelings, a guy who could be sensitive, maybe I could have a relationship again, but men aren't like that out there." She went on to talk about her twenty years of prostituting and how sex and money was what it was all about. I pointed out to Tania that she said Jake was different, and, if he could be different, there might be other men out there who could be different as well. And Jake said, "My HIV gave me a perspective. It made me think about life. I know when you get the rejection, it's devastating, but you can't let that take you over; otherwise you give up your recovery."

Jake had given us a list at the beginning of the meeting of fifteen things one should think about when one is in trouble to help the recovery keep going. He always made copies of material he received from his recovery group and brought them in to the members. Tania said, "Number five is what it's all about. Number five really is the story." She went on to quote number five on the list, "Do you fear the unknown?" Theresa said, "That's what I'm afraid of—the unknown. If I lose my boyfriend, who's going to take his place? . . . But the trust issue has been broken now. It's really been broken. I have to give him telephone numbers now, so he knows where he can reach me any-time during the day. That doesn't feel right. I don't think I should be doing that." John said, "I don't think you need to leave numbers for him. The die is cast. The deed is done, and you have to deal with that now, and maybe it's not going to be possible to 'remake the relationship.' " Theresa said, "I feel stuck on stupid." Tania reminded Theresa that her boyfriend started it with the "bitch." "He dissed you. Now the way you handled it on the telephone, that wasn't very ladylike, but you were too upset to handle it any other way."

After some additional discussion, we went back to Theresa. Theresa said that she really tried to hurt him and she was still feeling badly about that. John said, "Didn't you really hurt yourself, Theresa?" She was quiet for a moment, and then said, "Yes, I did. I know I do some of this stuff. I just want some attention, any kind of attention, even if I have to screw myself. At least someone pays attention. . . . This is really hard to deal with in recovery." Tania said, "You know, you sound like you were a scorned woman." Theresa recovered her anger at that point and said, "I'm mad. I'm really mad at him because I let him interfere with my recovery. He has not been taking his recovery seriously. He goes to the groups and he talks the talk, but he doesn't walk the walk."

John asked, "What are you expecting in the relationship? Maybe you're expecting too much. Maybe it's a waste of energy. Maybe you're setting yourself up to fail." Theresa said, "I have to give time, time." Tania said, "Look, if it's not going to work out, isn't it better that it happened now, instead of after five years? I know it's painful." John agreed with Tania that, if they were going to break up, it was better to do it now, rather than later. Theresa said, "I had high expectations," and then she began to cry. "I was getting sober. . . . I was okay. I was dealing with my problems. I didn't need another man. I was having fun with friends. I had girlfriends, people I could talk to, but I just didn't give time, time." John told Theresa that she had a lot of mixed feelings right now—the stress, the anger, a lot of negative energy. He wondered whether she shouldn't be careful in the next few weeks as she tried to make a decision about what to do next.

Theresa said, "It would be a lot easier if it wasn't the holidays. The holidays make it so much harder." Tania said, "Look, you were honest, you respected yourself. You may not have handled it well, but you were being grown up." Theresa said, "Maybe I didn't give it enough time. Maybe I should have waited a bit, 'cause he told me he loved me. He told me he was going to buy a ring and that he wanted to marry me." I pointed out that there was at least a possibility that he may have been trying to hurt her back when he said that.

Tania and others in the group agreed. Theresa said, "I felt violated by this guy." John asked what she was going to do over the holiday. She said she was going to go see her baby girl, and she had bought her a present, a little bracelet, which she has to get fixed for her. (Her child had been taken away by the Department of Social Services to live with a grandmother.) Theresa continued to cry and said, "I need some answers. What should I do? What should I do? You have to tell me what to do." John said, "No one can do that, Theresa. You will have to decide what to do yourself."

I asked Theresa how she was going to get through the next week or so. She said she was going to meetings regularly, and her sponsor had been really helpful. And then she turned to Tania and said, "And I can call you if I need to, can't I?" Tania said, "Anytime, anytime. I feel a lot of love and respect for you, and I would do anything I can to help you get through this." Jake said, "You can call me too." Theresa said, "I tried, but I couldn't get through." Jake said he turned his phone off from incoming calls, because sometimes he just wanted to be alone. I said to Jake that, if he did want to connect with other people, he'd have to turn his phone back on again.

The group meeting came to a close at that point. Theresa seemed more at peace when she left. I continue to feel that the mutual aid is building in the group and that the members are learning how to construct nonexploitive and caring relationships.

CONCLUSION

So what have I learned from this experience of crossing boundaries? I have learned to have more respect for other models of helping and to be prepared to draw upon them when they are appropriate for different populations. I have continued to learn how important it is for me to cross the town-gown boundary and infuse my teaching and my writing with direct contact with clients. I have seen the powerful way in which clients who are so different in so many ways can cross their own boundaries as they reach out to one another in aid of their mutual recovery and their struggle with a powerful and deadly illness. And, most of all, I have learned once again how resilient our most damaged clients can be, the incredible strength and caring they can demonstrate when we provide the medium of a mutual aid support group and help them use it to help one another. They were truly inspirational for me and I hope for you as well.

REFERENCES

Alcoholics Anonymous (1984). Pamphlet. New York: Author.

Bennis, W.G. and Sheppard, H.A. (1956). A theory of group development. *Human Relations*, 9(4), 415-437.

Bion, W.R. (1961). Experience in groups. In *Experiences in Groups and Other Papers*. London: Tavistock Publishers.

Fidele, N. (1994). *Relationship in Groups: Connections, Resonance and Paradox*. Wellesley, MA: Stone Center Papers.

Googins, B. (1984). Avoidance of the alcoholic client. *Social Work*, 29(2), 161-166.

Hardesty, L. and Greif, G.L. (1994). Common themes in a group for female IV drug users who are HIV positive. *Journal of Psychoactive Drugs*, 26(3), 289-293.

Matano, R.A. and Yalom, I.D. (1991). Approaches for chemical dependency: Chemical dependency and interactive group therapy: A synthesis. *International Journal of Group Psychotherapy*, 41(3), 269-293.

Prochaska, J.O. and DiClemente, C.C. (1986). Toward a comprehensive model of change. In *Treating Addictive Behaviors: Process of Change*, W.R. Miller and N. Heather (Eds.). New York: Plenum Press.

Schwartz, W. (1961). *The Social Worker in the Group: The Social Welfare Forum*. New York: Columbia University Press, pp. 146-177.

Shulman, L. (1999). *The Skills of Helping Individuals, Families and Groups*, Fourth Edition. Itasca, IL: F.E. Peacock Publishers.

Chapter 3

Where Has Real Group Work Gone? Reasserting the Fundamentals

David Ward

As the theme of this book is "crossing boundaries," I propose to examine what is happening to group work in Great Britain and consider what responses might be appropriate. I ask North American readers to decide for themselves what might be the connections with their practise in their different organisational and cultural circumstances.

To set the scene, I propose to recall a personal story, an experience which drew starkly to my attention some fundamental questions about the nature and place of the discipline which provides the common ground and link among the members of AASWG. Early in 1997, I was asked to write a chapter on group work for a new general textbook for social work students (Adams, Dominelli, and Payne, 1998). Initially, I thought this would be quite straightforward, but on thinking about possible content, I hit upon a problem. When I looked at work settings in which most of the text's readers would undertake their field practise and eventually work, I realized that group work had become all but invisible. When I scanned contemporary British professional literature, I found this omission substantiated. Following an outpouring in the 1970s and 1980s, the output on group work today is scant and, where it exists, is set at the margins of social work practise.

To contextualise this, it is necessary to say something about the organisation of social work in Great Britain. In Britain, social work is dominated by what we call "statutory responsibilities." These are legal duties placed mainly on municipal authorities for the protection of children, the management of the mentally ill and offenders, and practical services to the elderly and disabled, which are implemented in the main by social workers. Historically, most of this work has been contained within the municipal departments, although recently the grip of the public agencies has been weakened through market testing of welfare services and separation of purchaser and provider functions, bringing about an expansion of the "voluntary" and commercial sectors in social services. One result of this context is that, in Britain, the method specialisms have always been weak. Work with individuals dominates but is not called casework because of the association of that term with psychodynamic approaches. Community organisation has always sat outside mainstream social services, and, therefore, social work and group work has existed as an "add on," an optional extra to individual work. As such, group work has always been marginal, although in the 1970s and 1980s it was quite fashionable. However, swingeing cutbacks in the 1990s refocused practise on meeting legal duties and, with this, an individualised approach.

To return to my story, I quickly concluded that I could not, in conscience, provide a summary outline of group work theory and guidelines for practise. To do so would be to lose touch with the reality of the field and would render it subject to the frequent criticism of students that their texts do not connect with what they find in practise. Instead, I fell back, as I invariably do when confronted with a problem, on the process of self-directed group work (Mullender and Ward, 1991) for addressing problems. I decided to draft a contribution asking these questions:

> What has happened to group work?
> How should we respond?

WHAT HAS HAPPENED TO GROUP WORK?

- Group work has shifted to work *in* groups.
- The group as the *instrument* of change has shifted to the group as the *context* for intervention.
- Concern with the dynamics of the group *encounter* has shifted to a pedagogic *instructional* orientation.
- And, maybe by default, *democratic* and *collective* values have shifted to *authoritarian* and *individualistic* values.

Over recent years there has been a discernable trend towards groups that are increasingly task oriented, with decreasing emphasis being paid to process, reducing group work to a sterile exercise in which members receive packaged programmes that do not recognise them as unique individals often caught up in oppressive social conditions of poverty. Little, if any, attention is given to group dynamics and group work skills and methods.

These characteristics are particularly visible in the group-based cognitive behavioural programmes now in wide use in Great Britain, reflecting what Konopka (1990) describes as one-to-one treatment with the rest of the members acting as bystanders (cited by Kurland and Salmon, 1993, p. 8). Writing about work with male sex abusers, Cowbum and Modi (1995), two British practitioners, see in such approaches oppressive Eurocentric and heterosexist assumptions, grounded in conformity and obedience, but in fact potentially dangerous in reinforcing abusers' minimalist views of their own responsibility and the harm their actions have caused.

These changes can be contextualised within wider sociopolitical and economic changes that impacted social work in the 1980s and 1990s. A new ideological climate in which it is possible for a British prime minister to claim that "there is no such thing as society," the introduction of market practices to the delivery of social services, "new managerialism" as a drive towards client/user specialisms, the emergence of the law as a key defining factor, and new "competency-led" approaches to social work education and training have made it unfashionable and difficult to own many of the values and purposes of group work, which stress that

- the core process of group work is the interaction among a group of people based on mutuality as the means of achieving group purpose; and
- group work is antioppressive in its context purpose, method, group relationships, and behaviour (Brown, 1996, p. 83).

Group work may have become unfashionable precisely because it acknowledges that groups develop lives of their own, over which the workers cannot ever have complete control. In a group, the agenda is likely to be holistic and the process democratic. Groups members will raise issues that are important and significant to them, no matter what "ground rules" and boundaries have been set. Such free-flowing characteristics are out of kilter with the current climate, emphasising as it does discipline and individual responsibility and, at an organisation level, preset objectives and audited outcomes. The outcome is many projects and workers for whom the ideas of real group work are unfamiliar or, even worse, are regarded with suspicion.

HOW SHOULD WE RESPOND?

I think we have a problem with Anglo-American traditions. At root they are competitive and individualistic and in conflict with what we believe in. However, Brown (1996) identifies three key considerations for the future of group work: values, practise-based model building, and sustaining group work and group workers into the millennium (p. 90). What I would like to propose now is a practical reassertion of group work that can encompass these considerations.

A recent briefing by the National Institute for Social Work (1996) in Britain highlights that a major cornerstone for social policy, and a challenge for social work in the new enlarging Europe, is the fight against social exclusion. It argues that the challenge of reducing social exclusion demands new approaches to individuals and groups currently denied access to employment or services.

In this context we need to return to the historical connection between group work and equality and democracy. In my work with colleagues in Europe, east and west, I am inspired when I discern in other countries and cultures where mass unemployment, demographic changes, and the apparent inability of governments to sustain their welfare provision have created various forms of social exclusion, conscious efforts are being made to reframe welfare services in ways that enhance an inclusive group-orientated approach. In contrast, in the United Kingdom, we barely have begun a "facilitation" style of group work engendering an atmosphere of equality, enabling the women "to explore the humour, sadness and strains of family life and no longer remain silent about these" (Butler, 1994, p. 178). Central to the group agenda emerged structural dilemmas facing members: Women's sexuality and relationships with male partners were entangled with the processes of racism and the difficulties of bringing up mixed-parentage children. Faced with relentless hardships, the women easily identified the politics of poverty. Unpacking structural and individual issues was critical to these women's empowerment and the creation of their own solutions to the threats and dilemmas they faced (Butler, 1994, p. 163).

In the completely different setting of a young offenders' penal institution, Badham (1989) and colleagues worked with the inmates to develop a through-care service that the young men would see as useful and relevant by enabling them to raise issues and complaints within the institution and to prepare themselves for release. The workers sought to draw out of the young men, and to provide opportunities for them to learn, skills and knowledge that would help them survive both "inside" and after release. Confronting racist and sexist attitudes was part of this, and the worker team included women and black workers. The young men controlled the group's programme, producing, amidst wide-ranging discussions, advice booklets and arranging speakers on welfare rights, housing, parole, and temporary release. For invited speakers, including the governors, the group prepared their briefs, organised invitations, and devised questions so that they acquired the information they wanted. The governor acknowledged the value of the forum and saw in this different context hitherto unrecognised capacities in these inmates. One young man said on leaving the group, "It made you feel as though you can do something with your life while you are inside" (Badham, 1989, p. 35).

This then is the shape of a group work practise designed to tackle the processes of exclusion. Such group work is at its heart democratic and empowering; such group work has a place at the heart of democracy and empowerment. Of course, we must not be complacent nor uncritical, but, within group work, there are fundamentals which are sound, of which we can be proud, and which we must strive to recapture and reown.

REFERENCES

Adams, R., Dominelli, L., and Payne, M. (Eds.) (1998). *Social Work: Themes, Issues and Critical Debates*. London: Macmillan.

Badham, B. (Ed.) (1989). Doing something with our lives when we're inside: Self-directed group work in a youth custody centre. *Groupwork*, 2(1), 27-35.

Breton, M. (1994). On the meaning of empowerment and empowerment oriented social work practice. *Social Work with Groups*, 17(3), 23-38.

Brown, A. (1996). Groupwork into the future: Some personal reflections. *Groupwork*, 9(1), 80-96.

Butler, S. (1994). All I've got in my purse is mothballs! The Social Action Women's Group. *Groupwork*, 7(2), 163-179.

Butler, S. and Wintram, C. (1991). *Feminist groupwork*. London: Sage.

Cowbum, M. and Modi, P. (1995). Justice in an unjust context: Implications for working with adult male sex offenders. In Ward, D. and Lacey, M. (Eds.), *Probation: Working for Justice*. London: Whiting and Birch.

Konopka, G. (1990). Thirty-five years of group work in psychiatric settings. *Social Work with Groups*, 13(1), 13-16.

Kurland, R. and Salmon, R. (1993). Groupwork versus casework in a group. *Groupwork*, 6(1), 5-16.

Mullender, A. and Ward, D. (1991). *Self-Directed Groupwork: Users Take Action for Empowerment*. London: Whiting and Birch.

National Institute for Social Work (1996). *Social Exclusion, Civil Society and Social Work Briefing*. No. 18. London: NISW.

Chapter 4

Group Field Consulting: Building a Learning Community

Ellen Sue Mesbur

INTRODUCTION

This chapter describes a pilot project in group field consultation undertaken by the School of Social Work at Ryerson Polytechnic University in Toronto, Ontario. The project, implemented during the spring semesters of 1996 and 1997, involved third-year BSW students and their field instructors, all of whom were engaged in block field placements. The impetus for a new model of field consultation was initiated by two faculty members, both with many years of experience in field education and an interest in developing a model incorporating social group work with adult learning principles. Group field consultation was viewed as a medium for the development of mutual aid among students, field instructors, and faculty field consultants; for the promotion of diverse learning experiences; and as an innovative way of using field consulting time.

Feedback from students and field instructors demonstrated that the group approach was a positive experience and contributed significantly to an enriched learning experience. Shared perspectives were synergistic in nature, students were provided with the required support and opportunities to develop peer consultation skills, field instructors shared ideas regarding field teaching, and faculty field consultants were able to focus on student learning in an integrated manner.

DEVELOPMENT OF SUPERVISION
AND FIELD INSTRUCTION IN SOCIAL WORK

Individual Tutorial Models

Field education in social work has long relied on a primary model of field instruction that places individual students with individual field instructors, with a faculty field consultant/liaison usually assigned through the school. This tutorial or mentor model of supervision (Gitterman and Miller, 1978; Marshack and Glassman, 1991; Rabinowitz, 1987; Richard and Rodway, 1992) has characterized social work practice and social work education since the beginnings of the profession.

Early developments in social work supervision in both agencies and schools of social work paralleled early professional progress in that a psychoanalytical/casework model became a central feature of the supervision structure. This structure was characterized by individual supervision and mirrored many aspects of the worker-client relationship. Within this relationship, the supervisee (worker or student) was expected to focus attention on his or her feelings, self-awareness, personal insight, as well as transference and countertransference issues (Kaplan, 1988).

Multicomponent Models

The 1950s and 1960s saw a shift in emphasis in social work supervision toward a multiplicity of supervisory components: institutional, methodological, psychological, and educational (Kaplan, 1988). Getzel, Goldberg, and Salmon (1971, p. 159) proposed changes in supervision that included an emphasis on assistance through lateral relationships; increased accountability; greater exploration of difficulties through the use of the group structure; and the empowerment of students or workers. This model, initially created for staff development, moved

> the educational process of the entire agency away from a supervisory model grounded on a casework framework to an interactional or role systems one, noting that participation in group supervision hastens the development of practice skill and the

flexibility necessary for effective work. (Marshack and Glassman, 1991, p. 88)

Group Supervision Models

As early as 1942, Bertha Reynolds developed a framework for educating social workers, utilizing "group methods that relied upon principles of stage theory in group and educational development" (Marshack and Glassman, 1991, p. 88). Miller (1977) proposed the inadequacy of the casework perspective for group work supervision. He suggested that group work's distinctive intellectual and social traditions, with roots in progressive education and a milieu approach to service, contributed important knowledge about the supervision process.

New themes and interests operationalize the transition in the process and structure of supervision when group supervision emerged, particularly in the 1970s and 1980s, as a viable alternative to individual supervision. Miller (1977) concluded that growing interest and experimentation with the use of consultation, peer group supervision, team supervision, and various group methods of supervision could supplement or substitute for the traditional and primary technique of the individual conference (as cited in Getzel and Salmon, 1985, p. 29).

The educational component of supervision, although acknowledged from the beginning of social work history, also took on a greater emphasis in the 1970s (Getzel and Salmon, 1985). Gitterman and Miller (1978) declared:

> We cannot afford to permit the contemporary tendency to emphasize self-defined need for self-expression and self-actualization to transcend the content to be mastered or the task at hand that needs accomplishment. The process of education must not be removed from the substance of education. . . . Real learning takes place when the interaction or process is essentially a structured goal-directed activity in pursuit of substance and competence. (as cited in Getzel and Salmon, 1985, p. 35)

Getzel and Salmon (1985) acknowledged that "Group supervision . . . as the medium for bringing about conceptual change in people's lives brings it closer to the natural way in which people change and grow" (p. 31). In agency group supervision, the workers are generally accountable to the supervisor, with the supervisor assuming disproportionate responsibility for the functioning of the group (Abels, 1978; Shulman, 1982). "In peer group consultation, the group is composed of workers who occupy equal levels in an agency hierarchy or positions of similar description from different agencies. . . . Responsibility for the operation of the group is shared equally among all members" (Steadman, 1997).

Marshack and Glassman (1991) brought the concept of group supervision to the arena of field instruction:

> Group field instruction is closest to group supervision in interactional processes, affective intensity, and the supervisors' role. However, unlike the supervisor of professionals, the field instructor is required to help students in their struggle to integrate perspective on the professional role and practise technology. (p. 88)

As a primary method of field instruction, group field instruction promotes the notion of the effectiveness of social work groups as learning systems that enhance the processes of mutual aid, consensual validation, and feedback (Marshack and Glassman, 1991, p. 89). Kaplan (1991) noted:

> The theoretical underpinnings for group supervision stem from social group work theory. The concept of mutual aid (Shulman, 1982), i.e., that the sharing of data, the availability of lateral help, providing the arena in which sensitive issues may be raised, the support afforded through the awareness that members share similar concerns and the overall emotional support provided all augur well for use of this modality. (p. 142)

The Faculty Liaison Role in Field Education

The actual role of the faculty liaison in field education has garnered little literary attention, but certain developmental themes are evident: the liaison "linkage" function; the notion of a "faculty advisor," "faculty representative," or "faculty consultant" who performs advisory, educational, and administrative tasks with agencies and field instructors; an educational integrative function; and a multiple role function including evaluation of student progress, education of field instructors, integration, communication, and linkage (Raphael and Rosenblum, 1987, as cited in Fortune et al., 1995).

In the third part of a study of the liaison role, Brownstein, Smith, and Faha (1991) found lack of uniformity in the perceptions of the faculty liaison's role among schools, field instructors, and faculty liaisons. However, agreement existed on the liaison's perceptions of the roles of a mediator and a consultant. The authors suggested that further inquiry into the liaison's role is required in order to strengthen the partnerships between schools and agencies.

Fortune et al. (1995) reported on a study that compared field instructors' perceptions of the liaison role of two different models, the intensive model and the trouble-shooting model. In the intensive model, the liaison is actively involved in the educational experiences in the field and is central to the management of the practicum. In the trouble-shooting model, the liaison's contact with field instructors and students occurs only when difficulties arise and in which case intensive supports are mobilized to resolve the problem situation. Findings indicate that field instructors working with distinctly different field liaison models agree on many essential elements of the field liaison function. When differences occurred, "each group of field instructors expressed preference for elements of their school's Model: what they receive is what they prefer and what they consider important" (p. 291). Fortune et al. also noted that themes in literature identify the need for schools to take a "strong conceptual and educational role in monitoring and guiding the field practicum, through the field liaison role" (p. 291).

The relationship between schools of social work and their sponsoring universities with respect to the value placed on the field component of social work education has been fraught with tensions. Faculty members within the schools also place varying degrees of importance upon the field-consulting function. The few studies that have been conducted indicate that perceptions of the faculty liaison's role are mixed, with little agreement on the crucial elements of the role. If we accept that the role is inherently an educational one, then this purpose should guide our conceptualization of that role. Educational purpose will help us shape the field liaison's role and the manner in which that role is carried out. Schneck (1991) emphasized the educative role of the faculty as an "arbiter of change," one who mediates among the three representative groups in the field education experience: the students, the school, and the community. Teaching/learning activities in the field must be structured in such a way that the integration of learning is maximized (Norberg and Schneck, 1991). Norberg and Schneck noted:

> The answer seems to lie in the ability of students, agency instructors and faculty to consciously build the conceptual and experiential bridges between the students' field experience and learning needs, and the knowledge and skill resources wherever they lie. This can be accomplished through active, spontaneous, and non-possessive teaching/learning skills and activities. (p. 112)

THE GROUP FIELD-CONSULTING MODEL

The group field-consulting model was developed by two faculty members in the School of Social Work at Ryerson Polytechnic University as a means by which they could incorporate social group work with adult learning principles in the context of field learning. They were interested in enhancing the educational function of their roles as field consultants, in facilitating the necessary synthesis that must occur for students in their field education, and in developing an open climate for mutual learning among students, field instructors, and faculty. The model was composed of three elements: orientations, student integration seminars, and group progress reviews (see appendix).

Implementation of the group field-consulting model began in 1996 with two faculty field consultants, thirty-five students, and thirty-five field instructors, all of whom were involved in block field placements. In 1997, thirteen students and twelve field instructors participated in the group consultation model with one faculty field consultant. The block field placement required students to complete 364 hours per year in an agency, either three, four, or five days a week.

Orientations

Separate orientations were held for students and field instructors. Although both focused on the basic elements of beginning a field placement, the student orientation placed more emphasis on issues and concerns regarding getting started in a field placement and how to maximize the use of field instruction. Students were provided with handouts that included information on keeping a journal, developing a learning contract, writing a process recording, as well as the school's field education manual. As this was a first field placement for the majority of students, considerable time was required to adjust the students to the concept of experiential learning in an agency setting, the differences between being a worker and a student, the intensive experience in a block placement, and setting realistic learning goals. The group field-consulting model was presented and classified, and assurances were given that the faculty field consultants were also available on an individual basis for consultation with students, or with students and field instructors, should situations arise that might be uncomfortable to discuss in a group setting. A climate of mutual aid and support was established at this first session. The students who had already experienced a second-year field placement were able to contribute significantly to the orientation process and support those peers beginning their first field placement.

The orientation for field instructors was an opportunity to present the group field-consulting model and to discuss the various learning aspects of a block field placement, which differs from the longer, two-day-a-week placements that take place over two semesters (the model that is usually employed in the school). Many of the field instructors were experienced and had been with the school for a minimum of a year. However, few had previously supervised students in block field placements and none had participated in any form of group field consulting. Field instructors were given the school's field education manual as well as a special field instruction manual written by several faculty field consultants. The majority of field instructors responded positively to the group model, but a few remained skeptical and indicated their preference for the "old" one-on-one field consultation model. In the end, aside from those instructors restricted by the traveling time required to attend the group sessions, everyone agreed to participate in the group model, with the jury out on its efficacy!

Student Integration Seminars

The original intention of the faculty field consultants was to hold four student integration seminars over the period of the block placement. This time was to be counted as part of the students' hours for their field placements. Through consultation with the field instructors, it was decided that three seminars would be more realistic for the agencies, given that the placements were concentrated over a short period of time. In 1996, each faculty field consultant held the seminars for their respective students, with a participation average of sixteen students per seminar. In 1997, the thirteen students attended the seminars conducted by one of the faculty field consultants. Students were required to attend these seminars, even if their field placements were out of town. Field instructors agreed to give students the extra time needed to attend, recognizing that the seminars would enhance their learning process.

The content of the seminars was semistructured. Both faculty field consultants worked together to develop the curriculum but were flexible in adapting the content to the needs of the students that surfaced during the seminars. The first seminar addressed the general information presented in the previous student orientation and focused more specifically on the anxieties and issues students may have had during beginning stages of entering an agency and developing a learning plan for their field practicum. Attention was given to the field instruction process, to the use of journals, to process recordings and learning plans as pedagogical tools, as well as to specific practice issues students had begun to experience in their field placements. These same themes were incorporated into the 1997 seminars.

The second integration seminar focused on practice issues and on preparation for the upcoming group progress review. Interestingly enough, both faculty field consultants found that issues around personal values and ethical dilemmas emerged spontaneously in each of their groups during this session. A number of students had encountered situations that challenged them to reflect upon their values and the dilemmas presented to them through their field practicum. This led to a further discussion on one's development as a professional and the meaning this held for each student. Once again in the 1997 seminars, these themes were retained as content for the second seminar.

The final integration seminar dealt with the concept of termination with clients, with the agency, and with the field instructor as well as the use of the students and instructors as a learning group. The issue of socialization into the professional role continued as a topic of interest, as did evaluation of the seminars and the group field-consulting process (see appendix).

The Group Progress Reviews

At the initial field instructor orientation, a schedule for the group progress reviews was established. Each of the faculty field consultants divided their students and field instructors into two groups so that there would be no more than five students and five field instructors per session. Times were offered in the morning and the late afternoon to accommodate the different agency schedules. To avoid any difficulties, the same groups were maintained for the midterm and final progress reviews. For the 1997 group, times were again available for two groups, ensuring that the same groups were scheduled for the midterm and final progress reviews.

At the midterm progress review students and field instructors had an opportunity to talk about the agency, the various services offered, and the specific learning assignments undertaken by the students. The field instructors shared how they engaged in the field instruction process and presented their assessments of each student's strengths and areas for continued growth. Despite the fact that this particular constellation of participants was new, students had the support of other students and the faculty field consultant with whom they were already familiar, plus the field instructors knew one another and the faculty field consultant. Given the inherent risks and anxieties of any evaluation process, it was remarkable how easily the participants were able to engage in the group process. It was interesting to note that it was the students who took the lead in the beginning, having been given the choice at the start of the meeting. This set the tone for the field instructors and allowed for a safe yet very open level of discussion. Throughout the process, field instructors and students interacted with the entire group, which resulted in lively discussion and the exchange of feedback and ideas.

The final group progress review took place near the end of most students' field placements. As students had started at different times, and some were putting in more hours per week than others, the timing did not coincide exactly for all students. This did not, however, prove to be a detriment; to the contrary, it allowed those students closer to the end of their field placement to serve as an example for the others. In the review process, students and field instructors engaged in a discussion of the overall learning experience of the students' strengths and future learning objectives, as well as upon the experience of the group field-consulting model. There was overwhelming agreement that this model had been a positive demonstration of the development of mutual aid in learning. The additional element of sharing information about agency services and orientations to field instruction proved to be an unexpected outcome. For field instructors, this provided a valuable opportunity for networking and community building. Students appreciated hearing about their peers' practice strengths. They commented that the group approach took the "mystique" out of the evaluation process and rendered it much less threatening. Students and field instructors agreed that the group field-consulting model stressed the "process" of learning. Field instructors commented that the collaborative nature of the group field consultation provided them and their students with opportunities to "connect differently with one another." The group meetings also provided some structure for field instructors and students and helped focus them in their individual supervision sessions. For some students and field instructors, a missing element in the process was discussion with the faculty field consultant on some specifics regarding students' practice experience; however, process recordings and the student integration seminars provided the faculty field consultant and students with sufficient material to provide all participants a solid sense of the students' individual practice. Following up on the feedback from the 1996 groups which suggested that the model include one individual visit by the faculty field consultant, the 1997 group was offered the individual visit. Only one field instructor and student requested this encounter. Discussion with the 1997 group indicated that the individual visit should be built into the model by the school, rather than offering it as an option. All participants were overwhelmingly in favor of the school condoning the use of the group field-consulting model (see appendix). They felt that the model would lend itself to both the block and concurrent (two days a week over two semesters) field placements.

CONCLUSIONS

A collaborative effort in providing effective training to future social workers necessitates the involvement and integration of students, field instructors, and faculty. This integration can create an innovative opportunity that enriches the existing educational component in field placements by expanding on current conceptions of field instruction through the addition of a new entity to the constellation. That is, traditional field instruction includes two entities (student and field instructor) while the group field-consulting model includes four entities (students, field instructors, faculty, and group). The model incorporates the concepts from the social group work literature of a mainstream group, which is characterized by "common goals, mutual aid, and non-synthetic experiences" (Papell and Rothman, 1980, p. 7).

A group field-consulting model allows field instructors the latitude to question problems in conjunction with their students and, simultaneously, provides field instructors with varying degrees of assurance when confronted with problems into which they may have limited insight. A quintessential feature of this model is its ability to redistribute power, related to possession of knowledge, to students from field instructors and faculty, thus fostering in students independence, competence, and mature functioning.

The structure innate to a group field consultation model eliminates the field instructor as the "singular gatekeeper." This elimination is significant for students because it encourages independent, creative, and divergent thought as well as providing a more realistic replication of professional social work functioning. Simultaneously, group field consultation amplifies the positive results that have been elicited from the past transition to group supervision. Therefore, the inclusion of a group component in field education should hypothetically produce the following effects: additional lateral support; increased participation by students; stimulation of more relevant professional discussions; and, eventually, additional insights related to the inclusion of new perspectives.

The inclusion of the group in field consultation is intended to function as a catalyst for fostering broad, transferable social work skills. Integrated group field consultation parallels Matorin's (1979) redefinition of supervision: "Supervision should perhaps be redefined as helping students discipline their thinking and exercise their problem solving abilities. Students so supported might be better prepared for the demands of autonomous practise" (p. 152). Thus, the model should provide additional lateral support to all parties involved in field education. Faculty field consultants experience a situated opportunity to educate students; field instructors benefit from the additional support with regard to their educational responsibility; and students gain a multidimensional perspective of social work, as well as the additional lateral support of faculty.

Current societal realities present extraordinary challenges to contemporary social work practice, to social work education in general, and to field education curricula, processes, and structures in particular. As social, economic, and political forces are contributing to increasingly complex and critical needs of our community and as the social service system is rapidly transforming under these pressures, schools of social work must respond with innovative and creative structures and processes in the delivery of their field education programs. The group field-consulting model is one way for schools to meet the learning needs of students and field instructors, and to build a truly collaborative learning community.

APPENDIX:
FIELD-CONSULTING METHODOLOGY
AND OUTCOMES

What the Faculty Field Consultants Did

- Organized and facilitated the two orientation sessions
- Organized and facilitated the three student sessions
- Organized and facilitated the two progress reviews
- Assured availability for individual consultation
- Read the process recordings and learning contracts as well as provided students with written feedback
- Requested that students maintain a daily journal to highlight their learning process and as material for discussion during the integration seminars
- Provided field instructors with a manual
- Provided students with written information regarding journal keeping

Group Approach to Field Consulting: Methodology

- Student orientation workshop to block field placement and group approach
- Field instructor workshop to block placement and group approach
- Two progress review group sessions with field instructors and students together, one midway into the field placement and one near the end of field placement
- Three student sessions between May and the end of June

Positive Outcomes of Group Approach to Field Consulting: The Student Integration Seminars

The student group sessions provided *students* with

- opportunities to discuss learning issues with fellow students;
- opportunities to share learning experiences and receive feedback from peers as well as other field instructors;
- opportunities for mutual learning about practice issues, agencies, and services in the community and different approaches to supervision;
- case discussions leading to the development of learning themes, e.g., professional roles, personal and professional values, ethical dilemmas, legal implications, and interdisciplinary work;
- integration seminars, which were useful because students were not attending class and the sessions helped integrate theory with practice; and
- support from other students, which reduced feelings of intimidation when sharing fears and concerns.

Positive Outcomes of Group Approach to Field Consulting: Field Instructors

The group approach to field consultation provided *field instructors* with

- a positive group experience with other students and field instructors;
- the perspectives of other field instructors, agencies, and students generated by various ideas about learning assignments and approaches to field instruction;
- assistance in adjusting to the "pace" of the block field placement (which is quite different from a twice-weekly concurrent placement);
- a greater appreciation of different students' learning patterns;
- an opportunity to learn about other agencies and services; and
- networking opportunities with other agencies, which enhanced their own professional practice.

Positive Outcomes of Group Approach to Field Consulting: Students

The group approach to field consultation provided *students* with

- a positive group experience with other students and field instructors;
- an expanded view of social work practice by heading different perspectives and approaches;
- more than one social work role model (presence of other field instructors);

- an opportunity to receive positive comments from other field instructors;
- an enhanced learning experience through the group compared to one-on-one sessions because it was less intimidating and other students were sharing similar concerns; and
- the validation of hearing about one's strengths from one's field instructor in a group setting.

Negative Outcomes of Group Approach to Field Consulting

Drawbacks of the group approach to field consultation were

- the reduced individual feedback from the faculty field consultant compared to the one-on-one sessions; and
- the lack of case-by-case discussions of each student's work in the group sessions.

REFERENCES

Abels, P.A. (1978). Group supervision of students and staff. In F.W. Kaslow and Associates (Eds.), *Supervision, Consultation and Staff Training in the Helping Professions* (pp. 175-198). San Francisco: Jossey-Bass.

Brownstein, C., Smith, H.Y., and Fada, G. (1991). The liaison role: A three phase study of the schools, the field, the faculty. In D. Schneck, B. Grossman, and U. Glassman (Eds.), *Field Education in Social Work: Contemporary Issues and Trends* (pp. 237-248). Dubuque, IA: Kendall/Hunt.

Fortune, A., Miller, J., Rosenblum, A., Sanchez, B., Smith, C., and Reid, W.J. (1995). Further explorations of the liaison role: A view from the field. In G. Rogers (Ed.), *Social Work Field Education: Views and Visions* (pp. 273-293). Dubuque, IA: Kendall/Hunt.

Getzel, G.S., Goldberg, J.R., and Salmon, R. (1971). Supervising in groups as a model for today. *Social Casework,* 52, 154-163.

Getzel, G.S. and Salmon, R. (1985). Group supervision: An organizational approach. *The Clinical Supervisor,* 3(1), 27-44.

Gitterman, A. and Miller, I. (1978). Supervisors as educators. In F.W. Kaslow and Associates (Eds.), *Supervision, Consultation and Staff Training in the Helping Professions* (pp. 100-114). San Francisco: Jossey-Bass.

Kaplan, T. (1988). A model for group supervision for social work: Implications for the profession. Unpublished paper. Garden City, NY: Adelphi University School of Social Work.

Kaplan, T. (1991). A model for group supervision for social work: Implications for the profession. In D. Schneck, B. Grossman, and U. Glassman (Eds.), *Field Edu-*

cation in Social Work: Contemporary Issues and Trends (pp. 141-148). Dubuque, IA: Kendall/Hunt.

Marshack, E. and Glassman, U. (1991). Innovative models for field instruction: Departing from traditional methods. In D. Schneck, B. Grossman, and U. Glassman (Eds.), *Field Education in Social Work: Contemporary Issues and Trends* (pp. 84-95). Dubuque, IA: Kendall/Hunt.

Matorin, S. (1979). Dimensions of student supervision: A point of view. *Social Casework,* 60, 150-156.

Miller, I. (1977). Supervision in social work. *Encyclopedia of Social Work* (pp. 1544-1550). New York: National Association of Social Workers.

Norberg, W. and Schneck, C. (1991). A dual matrix structure for field education. In D. Schneck, B. Grossman, and U. Glassman (Eds.), *Field Education in Social Work: Contemporary Issues and Trends* (pp. 96-121). Dubuque, IA: Kendall/Hunt.

Papell, C. and Rothman, B. (1980). Relating the mainstream model of social work with groups to group psychotherapy and the structured group approach. *Social Work with Groups,* 3(2), 5-24.

Rabinowitz, J. (1987). Why ongoing supervision in casework: An historical analysis. *The Clinical Supervisor,* 5(3), 79-90.

Richard, R. and Rodway, M.R. (1992). The peer consultation in group: A problem-solving perspective. *The Clinical Supervisor,* 10(1), 83-100.

Schneck, D. (1991). Integration of learning in field education: Elusive goal and educational imperative. In D. Schneck, B. Grossman, and U. Glassman (Eds.), *Field Education in Social Work: Contemporary Issues and Trends* (pp. 67-77). Dubuque, IA: Kendall/Hunt.

Shulman, L. (1982). *Skills of Supervision and Staff Management.* Itasca, IL: F.E. Peacock Publishers.

Steadman, P. (1997). Classroom supervision: A proposed framework for introducing group supervision to the social work classroom. Unpublished paper. Toronto, Ontario: School of Social Work, Ryerson Polytechnic University.

Chapter 5

Night of the Tortured Souls: Integration of Group Therapy and Mutual Aid for Treated Male Sex Offenders

Dennis Kimberley
Louise Osmond

The modern world is developing an almost mystic sense of continuity and interdependence of mankind—how can we make
this consciousness and unique contribution of our time into a
small handful of incentives which really motivate human con-
duct?

Jane Addams (1929)

INTEGRATING CONTINUED THERAPY
WITH SUPERVISED MUTUAL AID

This chapter describes a demonstration study project conducted
out of the School of Social Work of Memorial University of Newfoundland. It is not as much directed toward the treatment of "treated"
sex offenders, as it is to a group intervention model that was designed
and refined in practice to address the complex problem of meeting
both the needs for continued therapy as well as the ongoing need for
mutual support for treated male sex offenders. The "third level group"

This chapter is dedicated to two of the tortured souls whose deaths have diminished
us and whose struggles have enriched our souls.

project lasted for three years and served over twenty male sex offenders; it was part of a comprehensive community-based assessment and treatment model for adult male sex offenders, designed by Kimberley and Rowe,[1] that included three levels of group intervention, integrated with comprehensive biopsychosocial assessment, individual, couple, or family therapy. This report analyzes the conceptual and theoretical base for the group as well as some of the practice issues and outcomes associated with integrating therapy and mutual aid within a sociopolitical context that promotes monitoring and supervision of sex offenders.

The Tortured Souls

We define the group members as "tortured souls" in the sense that the combination of their life experiences as sex offenders and victims impacted all levels of their being, their identities, and their "self."[2] Tortured soul is a metaphor for an identity that is not only overcome by a sense of fundamental unworthiness ("I'm ugly and disgusting") but overtaken by a belief that this self, if disposed of, would make the world a better place. One of the tortured souls took his own life recently; one of the tortured souls used to try to get the police to shoot him because he "was too cowardly to do it himself." It is not surprising then that one of the goals in the two latter groups in our program was that of self-rebuilding[3] and, within that context, integrating the treated sex offender identity into the whole as opposed to having it be the defining characteristics of the self.

Public perception would probably lead to the conclusion that these tortured souls were so "tortured" by virtue of having served "hard time" in some of the most demanding penal institutions in Canada. Public attitude includes the statement by a Canadian politician regarding releasing sex offenders into the general population of the prison and letting other felons deal with them—presumably through brutality or murder.

The reality is that by the time the offenders had reached this advanced group experience, the members were dealing more with a combination of thoughts, feelings, and interpersonal relationships associated with living "the life sentence of being offenders for life and victims for life,"[4] while having their victimization minimized and denied, and their offending maximized. Some of the characteristics of group members as offenders and as victims are summarized below. Lest readers conclude that the authors are making excuses for offenders by acknowledging and addressing their victimization, it is important to consider that within our clinical population of male offenders, 95 percent or more had experienced unwanted and undesired sexual intrusion and/or sex abuse as children; of the female sex offenders with whom we have worked, all (100 percent) had experienced sex abuse as children.

In this ostensibly homogeneous group, members were heterogeneous with respect to sex offense history and offense cycle patterns associated with feeling "tortured"; their patterns included

- multiple rapes and other sexually assaultive offenses against women in "straight society" and/or men in prison;
- invitation to touch, multiple molestation, oral sex, and/or intercourse with unrelated female children or unrelated male children (pedophilia—nonincestual);
- invitation to touch, multiple molestation, oral sex, and/or intercourse with related female children or related male children (pedophilia—incestual);
- sibling sex and sibling incest of various patterns;
- multiple and "compulsive" paraphilic noncontact offenses against women, men, and children (such as nonphysically aggressive indecent exposure and intrusive voyeurism);
- paraphilic arousal by and sexual contact with animals;
- arousal by the fusion of sex and violence; and
- sexual arousal through aggression and violence.

Among the sexual victimization patterns experienced by group members and associated with feeling "tortured" were

- multiple unwanted sexual intrusion by a male and/or female sibling;
- multiple molestation and/or forced sex by a male and/or female parent;
- multiple molestation and/or forced sex by a male or female grandparent;
- multiple molestation and/or forced sex by a male or female relative—nonparent;

- multiple molestation and/or forced sex by a male and/or female stranger;
- molestation and/or forced sex by a teacher or youth group leader;
- same-sex molestation and/or forced sex;
- fusion of sex abuse and violence, or threat of violence;
- fusion of sex abuse and reception of affection; and
- fusion of sex abuse and reception of attention.

Other contributing factors to feeling tortured included personal, marital, familial, or societal response. Among these are included

- revivification of offenses and/or victimization;
- hypervigilence based on victimization and distrust of self;
- serious difficulties with trust, attachment, and bond;
- confusing and paradoxical responses to interpersonal relationships;
- loss of parental rights and contact with children;
- loss of marriage and/or partner;
- expulsion and/or scapegoating of offender by extended family or community;
- expulsion and/or scapegoating of offender as victim, by extended family or community;
- loss of access to paid employment or loss of employment once hired;
- rejection by potential heterosexual or homosexual partner; and
- unjust harassment and brutality by police or other officials of the state.[5]

Although one might typically define the groups as homogeneous, even up to the third level, the group members most often emphasized heterogeneity. The rapists most often considered child molesters ("diddlers") as "the worst of a bad bunch." Among the child molesters, those who were homosexual were singled out for homophobic attacks—a triple stigma. (Consider the following attack: "Anyone who can fuck a little kid in the ass is sick.") Of the rapists, those who were the most violent were defined by their peers as being more disturbed. This standpoint of heterogeneity shifted considerably as each internalized that the fundamental beliefs, attitudes, values, feelings, and interpersonal relationship patterns that supported their sex offending had much in common, even though they could emphasize behavioral differences as part of a defensive routine. By the end of treatment, most referred to one another as treated sex offenders and had come to respect that effective mutual aid was based on accepting what they had in common while appreciating their differences.

A PHILOSOPHY OF TREATING
AND SUPPORTING THE TREATED

Comprehensive Biopsychosocial Assessment

The community-based program designed by Kimberley and Rowe in 1990 applied the philosophy that sex offenders were treatable and that one of the outcomes of a comprehensive biopsychosocial assessment was a determination of readiness for treatment and suitability for group treatment. The assessment followed a social work paradigm and, normally, was more holistic than standard psychological assessments, most of which used cognitive-behavioral or personality assessment paradigms. The biopsychosocial assessment was used to guide the group leaders in creating individualized strategies to meet individualized needs and to establish personalized goals. The collection of assessments typically provided guides to the project directors and group leaders in establishing group content and process, and in contracting with the members. All third level group members, except one, were assessed as treatable and as group ready. All but one had completed his treatment in at least one first level sex offender group. All but three had been exposed to a second level group. These men ranged in age from twenty-six to fifty-nine years old.

Pretherapy Psychoeducation

It is important to recognize that some of the sex offenders in our program had been exposed to a pretherapy psychoeducational group, operated under other auspices, before being assessed in the Memorial University Program. In such programs, typically, group members were exposed to information on sexual development and sex offending. The majority reported being exposed to highly confrontative strategies to "force" them to share information about their offenses and to "force" them to assume full responsibility for all their actions. Some evaluated these group experiences positively; some preferred a less confrontative or less informationally oriented group service; some evaluated their experiences as so confrontative and so controlling as to be a form of institutionally sanctioned emotional abuse. In short, some clients in our program had predigested notions of what they liked and what they did not like about group process and content; these issues became a common theme as the group developed.

First Level: Psychosocial Focal Group Therapy

The first level group therapy, in our program, while it had some psychoeducational components, was semistructured. It utilized many experiential exercises that enabled the offenders to reduce their defenses and to express their thoughts, feelings, and experiences, as well as learn to become effective "group citizens." In addition to having a social work focus on a population at risk, it had some elements of a focal group model: creating structure; targeting the issue of the sex offending and relapse prevention; being more goal-oriented; valuing the efficiency of structured experiences to encourage rapid change; and fulfilling a clear psychosocial educational function.[6] It was what we termed more "psychosocial educational," in that both offense-related information and control skills were learned, but so were attitude change, group process, and interpersonal relationship skills. Part of the plan was to give group members a common baseline; the importance of this was evident once group members moved on to more advanced group therapy (level two group) and structured mutual aid (level three group). Of significance was the fact that the large majority of this second level group were still on probation or parole.

The third level group could be defined as being composed of "treated sex offenders" because in the first level group the outcomes noted for most members were acknowledging the sexual offenses for which they were convicted; acknowledging responsibility for their sex offending actions, including those which were part of their offense pattern; learning about their deviant arousal patterns; learning not to use contributing factors to minimize responsibility for their offenses; increasing awareness and appreciation of the impact on their victims; moving toward genuine victim empathy; understanding their psychosexual development in relation to both their offenses and their own victimization; and internalizing norms that defined their offense-related actions as unacceptable and hurtful.[7] Those group members who moved on to a second level, more flexible and process-oriented group used a graduation metaphor and correctly viewed the second level group as a continuation.

Second Level: Unstructured Dynamic Group Therapy

The second level group therapy was more dynamic and less structured than the first level.[8] It utilized more the unstructured therapeutic process model, though it had some structured experiences and continued with some psychosocial education when needed—integrating process learning with content learning. Whereas the first group typically lasted twelve to sixteen weeks, the second level group lasted twenty-five to thirty weeks and included some sessions that were more like marathons. The second level group built on group citizenship skills[9] and enabled members to develop more trust, openness, genuineness, interpersonal relationship skills, and feelings of safety. They were then able to explore in more depth the dynamics of their sex offending behavior. They could move beyond thinking and behavior to affect; interpersonal relationship patterns; attitudes toward women, children, and men; fantasies and desires; dynamics of power and control; situational stressors; and issues of identity and identity management—the beginnings of self-rebuilding. Members were encouraged to explore their own victimization in depth and, within this context, to enrich their victim empathy. The group modeled more "constructive confrontation"[10] of members by others as opposed to the aggressive confrontation often modeled in sex offender treatment. Given the more dynamic nature of the group process and the depth of movement, those "graduating" to the third level, *structured mutual aid and interactional group therapy* were, in terms of both exposure and gains, treated sex offenders.

Third Level Group: Supervised Mutual Aid and Interactional Therapy

The Philosophy of Lifelong Vulnerability and Self-Monitoring

Having completed one or two levels of treatment, many of the sex offenders arrived at the same conclusions that had been reached in establishing the program:

- Sex offenders feel vulnerable and at risk of reoffense, probably for life.
- Effective relapse prevention sets the stage for more substantial treatment; it does not represent the final outcome of treatment or the end of need for help with support, risk control, and constructive change.
- Forty weeks in one's life are not sufficient to erode the impact of "living with a tortured soul"; one continues to live with offender and survivor issues for life.
- The problems of everyday life, in the "here and now" and anticipated in the future, must be coped with effectively and, if not addressed, may be associated with regression and a return to higher risk.
- Multiple levels of support in everyday life are needed even when group therapy was not in session or was not offered.[11]

The result was that an estimated 90 percent of the graduates of two offerings of the first two levels of group, as well as others referred from other programs, decided to enter into a group that combined mutual aid goals with advanced therapeutic goals.[12]

Within this context one could argue that the clients had become group dependent (pathologizing their needs) and that they had problems with termination. In contrast, our position is that members had *grown to recognize the value of interdependence* in meeting life's challenges. This pattern is not surprising given that the second level group was quite dynamic; consistent with Shulman and Page and Berkow,[13] the value of interdependence was supported and modeled.

The demonstrated value of interdependence is one of the reasons many members gave for making a commitment to the supervised mutual aid group. Some members offered their own reflections on interdependence, associated with both second and third level group experiences; they articulated the following themes: developing sensitivity to the problems and needs of others; becoming efficacious in giving support in a way that it is likely to be received; feeling safe in giving support without interpersonal control motives being dominant (an important transformation for the majority of sex offenders); learning to receive support while feeling more trust than apprehension; learning to act with reciprocity; feeling the strength derived from mutual collective action—often referred to as "pulling together"; feeling a sense of strength in the ability to attach and bond in a mutually supportive fashion. The mutual aid agenda was clear and accepted; the evidence for the latter was the degree to which members acted out mutual aid.

The third level group, with voluntary membership, was conducted successfully over three years. It had a core group of seven to eight members who came to most meetings and had up to twelve members; the core group was most active in the provision of mutual aid each to the other. While the group was being conducted and for three years thereafter, there was only one member who was actively investigated for reoffending; this parolee had committed his offense before his entry into the third level group. What follows is an analysis of the supervised mutual aid approach organized around some group practice-theory questions.[14]

GROUP PRACTICE IN INTEGRATING THERAPY AND MUTUAL AID WITH TREATED SEX OFFENDERS

Can group therapy balance the needs for personal and societal control in a high risk group with the demand that individuals undertake self-control?

The third level group emphasized the reality that, for most members, the risk of reoffending was variable and was a lifelong risk. Their group experiences had modeled responsibility taking, including the belief that one had the responsibility to protect self and others by controlling one's risks—sometimes interpreted as preventative actions. Internalizing interdependence norms enabled the development of more commitment to protect those at risk and to protect one another in the interest of self-protection and victim protection. The attitude was one of active prevention.

Paradoxical approaches are not new to social work. They have been used at least since the time that Otto Rank's work was in favor and the Functional School was in vogue.[15] In working with paradox to its advantage (functional paradox) the social group worker may take advantage of the dynamic so well expressed by Morrison (1983):

> Paradox lives and moves in this realm; it is the art of balancing opposites in such a way that they do not cancel each other but shoot sparks of light across their points of polarity. It looks at our desperate either/ors and tells us they are really both/ands— that life is larger than any of our concepts and can . . . embrace our contradictions.[16]

By the third level group, members had progressed sufficiently in their own growth, development, and transparency that paradoxical dynamics could be addressed at a conscious level. The narcissistic patterns of many sex offenders enabled them to understand self-protection. The paradox was that self-protection could be framed in such a fashion that potential victims are likely to be protected. From a mutual aid perspective, other members had the task of supporting those at immediate risk; victim protection through self-protection became a more shared responsibility. An example of such collective monitoring was the recommendation by the group that an incestuous pedophile openly discuss with his daughter the need for her to be present when he, now a grandfather, was in the presence of his granddaughter. This group member was helped in explaining to his daughter that his wish was to avoid hurting his granddaughter's feelings by leaving her presence, while ensuring that she was protected with respect to his risks. Other members recognized that they were becoming more aware of, and sensitive to, the feelings and needs of others, in part due to appreciating the risks and needs of one another.

Within the mutual aid process there was also a paradox in the dynamic that permits a sex offender to enhance potential victim empathy, as a self-monitoring and self-control strategy, by becoming more tuned in to the feelings of another sex offender—a group member who is expressing himself as a victim. The paradox is that it is through the eyes of the sex offender as victim that other offenders become more deeply in touch with the feelings of their victims; in turn, they are then more able to generalize to norms of pattern breaking for a potential victim with whom the offender might not otherwise empathize. Within this context, individual and group development with respect to the mutual aid dynamic of the group might be expected to model empathy for a potential victim of another member. An example was when one homosexual pedophile expressed empathy for the male child of a female friend who had come to trust another homosexual pedophile in the group; the constructive confrontation of the latter by other members was associated with the risk of a "breach of trust" and the potential impacts on the child, as well as recognizing the internal conflicts with which he, the group member, was living.[17]

Can group therapy balance the needs of addressing the issues of "here and now and everyday life" that contribute to risk while promoting mutual aid?

Social work has had a long history of promoting self-help and mutual aid. Since the time of Toynbee Hall and the YWCA movement, trained, volunteer, and paid leaders have facilitated mutual aid groups.[18] Classic mutual aid approaches promoted democratic ideals, mutual support, reciprocity, and self-actualization.[19] This group did not use the term "self-help" as it was agreed that it was best to differentiate from groups that do not have a professional coleader.[20] The group designed was not only mutual aid, it also deviated from the externally applied social control model in that it promoted democratic process and mutual support goals as well as the use of mutual aid and other group processes in the interest of social control goals.[21] This dialectic between freedom and control was a major and significant dynamic in a group in which most of the members were there voluntarily, and where there was a clear agenda of the lifelong self-control of risk as well as voluntarily becoming good group citizens.

What was complex about this group was that it had primary goals of maintaining risk reduction and control (a social control function) with that of mutual aid (a self-control and interdependent control function). There was a dialectic tension between internalized controls and externalized, or "other" based, controls. This dialectic was layered in that the leadership responsibility of the group therapists was reduced in the interest of enhancing the mutual aid effectiveness of the group members, but if the members did not act out mutual aid strategies in high risk areas, then the therapists would model consciousness raising or constructive confrontation strategies. The paradox was that men who were practiced in exercising interpersonal control strategies in the interest of victimizing were now put in the position of joining to exercise group "controls" in the interest of reducing risks to potential victims as well as their group members. This norm was internalized to such a degree that one man expressed that if he acted on his fantasies, he was not only letting himself down but "letting the group down." Group members affirmed that if he "failed," then they would feel that they had failed both him and the victim. In addition, group members developed insight to the point of enabling another member to reconsider the risks associated with an action, such as theft or infidelity, that were not directly related to the sex offense risk. The intensity of the social control dynamics exercised through group process and cohesion was evidenced when some members acknowledged that the commitment not to "let down" the group was sufficiently motivating to enable pattern breaking in earlier stages of their offense cycles. Within this context, the dynamic tension between internalized and externalized "self" controls acted in the best interest of protecting the group, in that mutuality of feeling resulted in a sense of responsibility for the failure of a member to protect a potential victim.

How can group therapists and leaders enable the development of mutual aid skills and responsibilities while maintaining some continued therapeutic function and leadership responsibility?

The cotherapists' functions included various levels of social group work. In addressing past issues that surfaced or new stressors in the members' everyday lives, therapeutic interventions were needed that typically went beyond the skills of group members to lead, in either evaluation of challenges or in initiating processes to enable change. Issues such as sexual dysfunction, addictions, psychiatric (mental health) problems, new offense risks, anger and violence risks, new traumatic memories of offenses or victimization (flooding), sibling incest experiences, or the stress of potential new charges normally required the group leaders to assume more control of the process—sometimes even structuring interactions through the use of grounding or psychodrama techniques. The basic strategy was to cue the members when the professionals were needing to take more control and to cue ourselves (group coleader to group coleader) when we could enable group members to resume more leadership. One example was "grounding" a group member who was experiencing a flashback and who felt a sense of panic that he would lose emotional control "and not be able to come back [to reality]."

Most often, group members would cue the coleaders when they needed more "therapeutic help." On the other hand, they would often initiate meetings on their own when the group leaders were not available. At times, the group members would identify a theme, requesting that the therapists take the lead in sharing expertise on a topic of current importance to many of the members (e.g., normative problems of intimacy and sexual expression after their own victimization). At other times, the group members would assume responsibility for a theme such as early pattern breaking in the offense risk cycle, based on their "expertise" in what they termed the "university of hard knocks."

Group development and progress evidenced therapeutic processes and content themes that were acted out while enabling the refinement of group membership skills such that most members learned to undertake more mutual support responsibilities. Within the group meetings, these men, who had generally presented themselves as tough, learned to show compassion, warmth, understanding, sensitivity, support, and to offer comfort.[22] Outside of the meetings, they learned first to "be there . . . to be able to be counted on," to share in another's pain without the need for expert therapeutic intervention, and to deal with crisis intervention and stress through mutual support and problem solving. The progress in balancing mutual aid and therapeutic responsibilities was dependent on the dynamics of transition from a second level group to the third level group, feelings of trust and confidence in one another, as well as months of sharing and protecting mutual confidences.

What dynamics were created when a female cotherapist joined a group of male sex offenders, a significant portion of whom had abused or assaulted women?

It is not uncommon for sex offender groups to have male and female cotherapists.[23] Besides providing group members with a female perspective, and modeling of male and female roles, the use of co-therapists enables men with generally negative and otherwise distorted attitudes toward women to observe more respectful and egalitarian exchanges between a man and a woman. What is significant in the mutual aid group is that the female cotherapist was operating in a context of group development where power and control were being "returned" to men who typically exhibit serious problems and misuses of interpersonal power and control dynamics.

The first dynamic that was acted out by many of the men was to employ strategies to test acceptance and to promote rejection. The cognitive script that the men eventually expressed was "How can she be with us and accept us knowing what we did?" In early sessions with a new female cotherapist, established professional or student, some of the men, even at the point of introductions, would describe their offenses in graphic detail. If the female coleader absorbed the shock in the first two to three group sessions, if she continued to express acceptance of and concern for the person, then she was accepted as "OK"—accepted as a group member. Lest the reader misjudge that these men were simply acting out the aggression and control that they felt toward women, it is important to consider that they typically took responsibility for the process of "initiation" and for their actions in relation to testing out the new coleader member—male or female. They demonstrated insight into the dynamic interplay between the need for acceptance and the belief that they did not have the right to be accepted or cared about; this was juxtaposed to the fear of rejection and the belief that "civilians" or nonoffenders had good reason to be rejecting.

Group members then typically moved to define the female therapist as an expert on female matters. They confirmed the importance to them of a woman's perspective and feelings about them, their behavior, and their progress. They also declared that they were becoming more comfortable and safe in sharing their genuine thoughts and feelings with a woman, in their own words (e.g., "That slut of a wife of mine is whoring around"). It appeared that empathy and positive regard from a female was highly valued by group members, including the homosexual and bisexual members.

The female therapist moved to more acceptance as a group member when the group responded to her expertise, beyond the stereotypical standpoint of "the woman's perspective." She was called upon, for example, to problem solve on more refined relapse prevention strategies, to help with problems of distress in disclosing offender status to potential new employers, or to assist in the process of apologizing to the offender's victim. In short, the female cotherapist appeared to gain more acceptance at the point that group members expressed confidence in her thinking beyond "female issues" and outside of the boundaries of "the female perspective."

Most significant, even more mutual trust was expressed at the point where group members accepted primary leadership from the female therapist. This happened because of strategy (less active response from the male therapist), as part of the natural group development process (as trust developed, more members would "look to" the female leader to help them get unstuck in a group process), and as a default reality when the female member decided to lead the group on her own when her cotherapist was not available. To the men, the latter was the most symbolic of mutual trust; that the female cotherapist felt relatively safe with them was a valued gesture and was taken as a concrete symbol of their progress.

Sexual dynamics of attraction and arousal present a complex issue. At this advanced level, group members had the ability to declare more openly their attraction to a female therapist. Their openness was respected and processed. The issue was not politicized but treated as normal. This response was appreciated, especially by men who had been marginalized from society and who had been excluded from intimacy and shared sexual expression, sometimes for years.

The politics of sex abuse by females was another significant issue that the group had to address, with the response of the female cotherapist being dominant. Of the men who joined the group, four had been sexually abused by one or more females: mother, grandmother, cousin, and baby-sitter. One had had a "consenting" sexual relationship with an older sister that was dynamically related to both his victimization as a child and to his offense pattern. Disclosure of the victimization and premature eroticization experiences, initiated by older girls and women, was most difficult for the men. It was important to them that a female could confirm and appreciate group members' experiences and pain associated with physical, emotional, and sexual abuse at the hands of women.[24] Within this context of mutual acceptance and trust, the female therapist was more able to join in enabling "treatment effect," including the development of group citizenship skills.

How do group members resolve political and therapeutic issues of treating the sex offender as both offender and victim in the same context?

From a mutual aid perspective there were two dominant issues with respect to the dialectic of relating to the offender as victim. On the one hand, members were offenders and could use their victimization as a defensive routine to escape dealing with the realities of their offenses, with respect to themselves or their victims. On the other hand, the offenders were all victims of either sexual abuse or physical abuse; they had issues of the past to address, as the feelings lived in the present and some experienced revivification of previously unrecalled trauma. As Shulman has described, the dialectic in the sex offender group paralleled or modeled the dialectic that members faced in society[25] as well as in a penal system where the politically correct response was to maximize offender identity and minimize victim-survivor identity in male perpetrators. The progress of members by the supervised mutual aid group was evidenced by the fact that members often confronted one another if there was any suspicion that their victimization was being focused upon for too long (the threshold being five to ten minutes). The group norm could be said to have been congruent with the intolerance in society toward male offenders, especially sex offenders. The paradox was that applying the social work dictum of "beginning where the client is," when that meant beginning with the offender as victim through the medium of supportive group process and mutual aid, could help serve one of the primary goals of risk control.

Paradoxically, at this more advanced level, it was through exploring thoughts, feelings, attitudes, and relationship patterns associated with their own victimization that members gained more insight into their own offense dynamics. The combination often enhanced genuine victim empathy (although some had to be confronted on their continued use of empathy in a strategic and narcissistic fashion). One example of dealing with victimization and staying with the client is a striking response in which a member recalled yet another of his victims and acknowledged other offenses, based on a cue that he revivified in his own victimization. It is significant that another member was encouraged to take responsibility for another offense and to apologize to the victim even though he recognized that the victim would then have evidence sufficient to support charges; he was supported by the group in this painful and anxiety provoking process of recalling details and acknowledging yet another set of offenses and victim (now an adult). In short, victim empathy, societal protection goals, and restitution goals may be reinforced by treating the offender as victim— with due respect to timing and defensive routines.

Can group process, including mutual aid, support family reunification goals for sex offenders?

Half of the sex offenders, and at times their families, entertained family reunification goals. The group process could be both facilitative and resistant with respect to the reunification goals. One of the dynamics that confounded the decision process was the rejection that over one-half of the members had experienced from their families. Mutual aid norms could be confounding in these situations. Consider the following strong positions taken by the group (paraphrased) in the interest of member support:

- It is not wise for you or the victim to return to live where the victim is living; it will hurt her and you.
- It is not a good idea for you to return to a marriage where your partner was active in victimizing your daughter and has not dealt with her issues as you have yours.
- It is best that you have no further contact with the daughter that you hurt because your ex-wife will cause trouble for both of you and will not let you and your daughter get back to a more normal life.
- If your normal and reasonable sexual needs are not going to be met in that relationship, then by going back you will be increasing your relapse risk.
- If your daughter is prepared to have you back in the home, she is old enough to take care of herself now, so it should work out, if your wife gets used to you being back.
- If your wife can live with the fact that you raped another woman, then it's good to go back; you could use the support.

- If your partner wants you back, even though her daughter will be taken into care if you go back, then you are stuck; either way someone loses.

It is obvious that each of these group member positions represents a complex issue. The cotherapist's role was to enable the group to consider other alternatives or variations of a theme. The mutual aid perspective emphasized that the member arrive at a decision that would work for him in his particular situation. The expectation was that he would then receive support in making his decision work, supported as long as other key stakeholders in the decision (e.g., expartner) participated in arriving at a decision. The group also took an active role in helping the member evaluate and control victimization and revictimization risks.

Can the group process, including mutual aid activities, support resocialization of men who have been institutionalized and marginalized?

The majority of convicted male sex offenders are rejected and otherwise marginalized, yet to maintain both treatment effect and risk control, resocialization and reintegration are most likely necessary. The group processes, both therapy and mutual aid, as well as some session content, enable most of the offenders to "move in" from the margins. In this respect, the group was often instrumental in enabling self or identity reconstruction of the responsible, nonoffending, protective, lower risk, and restitutive self. One example of the mutual aid process converging outside of the group is reflected in the following:

One member who had to deal with a psychiatric illness as well as his offenses, and who had been falsely accused of another offense, left a men's hostel to set up his own apartment. Some of the group members joined him in his new home and coached him on self-care and meal preparation. He began to assume the identity of someone who could take control of his own life without being so heavily medicated or so reclusive. Paranoidal ideation, depression, and anger were reduced by a combination of systemic change and effective use of mutual support. A follow-up visit by some group members resulted in reports that he was taking better care of his home and himself. In the group members' terms, he began "to get a life."

The process of enabling group members to become "good group citizens," through three levels of group, was normally paralleled by the member becoming more integrated into community life, family life, and/or extended family life.

How does the group respond to and integrate new members given an open group with periodic entry?

The first theory we applied for integrating new members did not work well. The leaders attempted to take new second level group members and third level group members and integrate both into what was metaphorically labeled "a new group." The third level group members were resentful in that they defined themselves as having graduated and progressed beyond the second level group. They also had developed an identity and cohesion associated with having been the first of what they treated as a noble social experiment—professionally "supervised" mutual aid for treated sex offenders.

The second theory, while neither generous nor equalizing, enabled the third level group to receive and integrate new members—on its terms. The mutual aid group interpreted that new members had "graduated" to a level of insight and responsibility for self; that a life-long commitment to risk control, self-development, and mutual support was possible; and that new members could be counted on to genuinely work at not letting either themselves or the group down. The group's interpretation enabled the successful integration of many new members who permitted themselves to become part of a group that had an established identity, rules, and power structure.

Why the focus on being good group citizens?

The sex offender treatment and group literature is dominated by a somewhat politically correct cognitive-behavioral model. This model supports more the significance of structure and content than it does process and affect. The net result is that a set of important opportunities for risk control and potential victim protection are lost. The process of learning to be "good group citizens" involves internalizing scripts that support empathy, sharing, responsibility, interdependence, care, bond, and a partially reconstructed identity. The act of being good group citizens sets the stage for generalization beyond group sessions and patterns of thinking and behavior that may be logically and directly linked to relapse risk. The emphasis on interpersonal process skills and competencies, some of which are linked with good citizenship, in turn, supports effective mutual aid. The process, membership, and interactional themes modeled in this mutual aid experience supported psychosocial stability, genuine change in attitude and affect, the maintenance of treatment effect, prosocial change and social integration, and identity transformation—all of which are representative of more substantive change than are modification of behavior and the change of "distorted thinking" alone.

A striking example of mutual aid and good citizenship in the sense of shared social responsibility was one man who was terminally ill, living in chronic pain, and on social assistance, who would travel two hours, at times under hazardous conditions, at his own expense, to attend weekly group sessions. Group members took a collection to help him with expenses. When he became less able, two members traveled to pick up their group member—a four-hour round trip. When he became hospitalized, group members visited him. When he died, some members attended his funeral. The group processed grief and loss and took strength from the resilience and the healing path of another tortured soul.

CONCLUSION

This chapter addressed issues of group development and articulated strategies and techniques that enable the achievement of personal therapeutic goals, group goals, and mutual aid strategies to support risk control, community safety, offender reintegration, and identity transformation. In our analysis we addressed group dynamic issues associated with a high risk and experimental group that was used for demonstration and professional development purposes. As support for this supervised mutual aid group ceased, members attempted to keep it alive as a mutual aid group only. It worked for a while, but members still had therapeutic needs to be addressed. The conclusion that we can make is that some succeeded more than others, few failed, and some had a combination of results. From a correctional point of view the group was a success, with only one of its members known to have reoffended in a five-year period.

No man is an island, entire of itself.
Every man is a piece of the continent, a part of the main.
If a clod be washed away by the sea, Europe is the less . . .
[So] any man's death diminishes me because I am
    involved in mankind.
And therefore never send to know for whom the bell
    tolls.
It tolls for thee.

John Donne
Devotions Upon Emergent Occasions (1613)

NOTES

1. M.D. Kimberley and W. Rowe (1992). *Training, Collegial Consultation and Network Support for Sex Offender Assessment: Therapy and Relapse Prevention.* St. John's, NF: Memorial University, School of Social Work. M.D. Kimberley and W. Rowe (1991). *Sex Offender Assessment and Treatment: Needs, Challenges and Strategies for Newfoundland and Labrador: A Position Paper.* St. John's, NF: Memorial University, School of Social Work. We wish to thank Correction Services of Canada and Memorial University of Newfoundland for their support of this project.

2. B. Bettelheim (1982). *Freud and Man's Soul.* New York: Random House.

3. For a discussion of self-reconstruction within the context of groups, see W.D. Stone (1992). The clinical application of self psychology. In R.H. Klein, H.S. Bernard, and D.L. Singer (Eds.), *Handbook of Contemporary Group Psychotherapy* (pp. 177-208). Madison, CT: International Universities Press.

4. This is a paraphrase of an expression coined by one of the offender-victims in the group.

5. In conducting professional training sessions on sex offender treatment we typically have the group process the feelings that they might have as group members having such characteristics and labels. We ask social group workers how they would process relating to other group members as both offenders and victims.

6. See, for example, P.H. Ephross (1997). Group work with sex offenders. In G.L. Grief and P.H. Ephross (Eds.) *Group Work with Populations at Risk* (pp. 175-187). New York: Oxford University Press. See also M. McKay and K. Paleg (Eds.) (1992). *Focal Group Psychotherapy* (pp. ix-xii). Oakland, CA: New Harbinger Press.

7. For an early example of a social group work program for sex offenders that incorporated many of the components found in the first and second level groups in our program, see K. Helde (1995). Sex offenders group treatment: The ESTAT experience in Toronto, Canada. In R. Kurland and R. Salmon (Eds.), *Group Work Practice in a Troubled Society: Problems and Opportunities* (pp. 177-188). Binghamton, NY: The Haworth Press.

8. R.C. Page and D.N. Berkow (1994). *Creating Contact and Choosing Relationship: The Dynamics of Unstructured Group Therapy.* San Francisco, CA: Jossey-Bass.

9. H.S. Flack (1988). *Social Work: The Membership Perspective* (pp. 185-193). New York: Springer Publishing.

10. For discussions of constructive confrontation, see R.R. Kurtz and J. Jones (1973). Confrontation: Types, conditions and outcomes. In J. Jones and W. Pfeiffer (Eds.), *The 1973 Annual Handbook for Group Facilitators* (pp. 135-138). LaJolla, CA: University Associates Press; and P.J. Flores (1988). *Group Psychotherapy with Addicted Populations* (pp. 279-320). Binghamton, NY: The Haworth Press.

11. For results of a study regarding what group members, within self-help, define as supportive, see R. Wuthnow (1994). *Sharing the Journey: Support Groups and America's New Quest for Community* (p. 170). New York: The Free Press.

12. L. Shulman (1992). *The Skills of Helping Individuals, Families and Groups* (Third Edition, pp. 273-283). Itasca, IL: F.E. Peacock. L. Shulman and A. Gitterman (1994). The life model, mutual aid, oppression, and the mediating function. In A. Gitterman and L. Shulman (Eds.), *Mutual Aid Groups, Vulnerable Populations, and the Life Cycle.* (Second Edition, pp. 3-28). New York: Columbia University Press.

13. Page and Berkow, *Creating Contact and Choosing Relationship*, pp. 18-23, 233-261; and Shulman, *The Skills of Helping Individuals*, pp. 9-16. For another perspective on the significance of interdependence in group process and society, see J. Anderson (1984). *Counselling Through Group Process* (pp. 201-216). New York: Springer Publishing.

14. Female graduate social work students as well as graduate professional social workers were given opportunities to work with treated male sex offenders through the groups within our program. Observational notes and questions were produced to enhance social group work education.

15. O. Rank (1936). *Will Therapy and Truth and Reality.* New York: Knopf.

16. M.C. Morrison (1983). In praise of paradox. *The Episcopalian*, January, as cited in K.K. Smith and D.N. Berg (1987). *Paradoxes of Group Life.* San Francisco, CA: Jossey-Bass.

17. It is important for the reader to keep in mind that most of the members of the supervised mutual aid group had completed all the terms of their sentences.

18. K. Reid (1983). The use of groups in 19th century England: Preface to the American experience. In N.N. Goroff (Ed.), *Reaping from the Field from Practice to Principle* (Volume 2, pp. 860-879) (Proceedings of Social Group Work Three—1981). Hebron, CT: Practitioners Press. See also J. Anderson (1997). *Social Work with Groups: A Process Model* (pp. 18-19). New York: Longman.

19. U. Glassman and L. Kates (1986). Techniques of social group work: A framework for practice. *Social Work with Groups*, 9(1), 9-13.

20. J. Lobdell (1983). Comparative evaluation of therapeutic self-help and conventional therapy groups. In N.N. Goroff (Ed.), *Reaping from the Field from Practice to Principle* (Volume 21, pp. 51-57) (Proceedings of Social Group Work Three—1981). Hebron, CT: Practitioners Press.

21. See a summary of these goals by G. Konopka (1972). *Social Group Work: A Helping Process* (p. 31). Englewood Cliffs, NJ: Prentice-Hall.

22. In the beginning, physical touch was very awkward for these men; homophobia was confronted by one of the homosexual members who led the group in a consciousness-raising constructive confrontation.

23. Helde, Sex offenders group treatment, p. 180.

24. Based on the question being asked in only one direction, there is the accurate but selective perception by some professionals that male sex offenders typically hate women; in our experience they have been hurt by men and hate men as well. Their crimes against women are the focus of attention; their crimes against adult males are largely dismissed. Unfortunately, too many of the female cotherapists experienced much more rejection from other professionals than they did from the sex offenders.

25. Shulman, *The Skills of Helping Individuals*, pp. 275-276.

Chapter 6

Pushing the Boundary
and Coming Full Circle:
A Contemporary Role for Social
Group Work in Service Education

Joanne Gumpert
Sue Burrus
John M. Duffy

As colleges and universities broaden their missions beyond equipping students with the academic skills to excel in their chosen careers, education for socially responsible citizenship, integrity, and cooperative team membership is increasing on campuses across North America. These goals are reached through a variety of service-oriented programs that take students out of the classroom and expose them firsthand to complex social problems and individuals who are attempting to hold their lives together as they cope with their impact. A recent Higher Education Section of *The New York Times* described programs at various institutions of higher education, such as Harvard University, the University of Denver, the University of Southern California, Emory University, and Marywood University, that reflect this current shift to community service as a significant means of educational instruction (Marriott, 1996; Niebuhr, 1996). This chapter focuses on one of these institutions and discusses a cooperative arrangement between the School of Social Work and Campus Ministry at Marywood University in which graduate social work students use social group work intervention to enhance the experience of undergraduate students who have volunteered to participate in Spring Break Service Trips to Appalachia.

As this project pushed the boundary for the use of social group work practice to include service learning, it came full circle to the very philosophical underpinnings that spawned the practice methodology being used. The settlement house movement, initiated in the late 1800s, was built on the belief that young college and university students could gain greater understanding about poverty and its associated problems by sharing the life experiences of the poor. In 1883 Samuel Barnett, the Vicar of St. Jude's in Whitechapel, East London, spoke at Oxford on the theme "settlements of university men in great towns" and called for the students to "join in sharing the life of that, to us, dim and strange other world of East London." In February 1884, Barnett opened Toynbee Hall, named for an Oxford History lecturer who had worked in East London, and Oxford students joined him at the first settlement house (Briggs and Macartney, 1984). Soon after, Jane Addams arrived at Toynbee Hall to see for herself Barnett's program and a year later, in September 1889, founded one of the best-known settlements in the United States, Hull House in Chicago. Rapidly, settlement houses opened in the major cities of North America and for over a century have provided university students with opportunities for many types of experiential education, or as Addams (1910) said, these students were "learning of life from life itself." The consonance of the underlying philosophies has eased the integration of social group work with service education.

In contrast to the earlier practice in settlement houses, where social workers dealt directly with those in need, in this endeavor, the group work intervention is focused on deepening the experience of undergraduate students in order to effect their awareness of social problems and attitudes about social justice as they engage in meeting basic needs of the poor. The following sections include a review of the relevant literature on service learning, a description of the field placements and the work accomplished, as well as a discussion of preliminary findings on the impact of this group intervention with undergraduate students engaged in service trips to Appalachia.

LITERATURE REVIEW

Essentially, service learning involves bringing students into the community face to face with others and themselves, and then bringing the reality of that experience back to the classroom. The literature on volunteering provides insight into the reasons students choose to participate in service experiences. Beginning with studies of the initial motivations of individuals who volunteer to help others, to studies looking at effects of specific service learning programs, research supports this balance of experience, service, study, and reflection, noting impacts of experiential education and service learning on the social, psychological, and intellectual development of the students who participate.

Much of the periodical literature on volunteers focuses on recruiting, training, and retaining volunteers in specific roles. Many volunteers do focus their efforts on a specific context or activity. It appears to be important to recognize their commitment to those specialized issues or segments of the community (Sundeen, 1992). Other research, however, explores broader issues providing a conceptual link between specific volunteer programs, studying the motivations that lead people to volunteer in particular programs, and relates to the broad developmental effects in social, psychological, and intellectual realms.

Categories of variables identified in looking at volunteer participation include *context,* referring to the environment of the individual, social group, or community; *social background,* referring to social status, role, education, and gender; *personality,* referring to general personal response tendencies such as extroversion or assertiveness; *attitudes,* referring to more situation-specific response tendencies; and *situation,* which refers to factors in one's immediate location or one's own definition of that environment (Smith, 1994). Smith goes on to note that volunteer participation is multidimensional and that understanding the dimensions involved in any one person's initial impetus to volunteer time and/or services is crucial for effective recruitment and in providing appropriate, adequate supervision, thus influencing whether a person will continue to volunteer.

The actual reasons that a person volunteers may not be obvious. People who work with volunteers in organizations that provide services to the terminally ill have found that to be able to work with their clients, these volunteers must be prepared to anticipate their own reactions to difficult client situations and to face their own personal grief and stress. They have identified five factors that are useful in understanding other volunteers also:

1. *Helper principle* refers to personal benefits received as a result of volunteer experiences. It seems to confirm actual, therapeutic gain made by helping others.
2. *Self-serving* represents a self-orientation to voluntarism, i.e., looking after oneself and taking care of one's own interest.
3. *Self-esteem* contains items explaining feelings of self-worth.
4. *Identification with the group* concerns the degree of comfort the volunteers have with sharing their volunteer association with others.
5. *Power* has an underlying theme related to the volunteer's need for power and control. It is interesting to note that the research suggests that many types of volunteer activities "provide the individual with opportunities to influence, direct, or control the lives of others" (Schondel, Shields, and Orel, 1992).

With the exception of *power,* the factors identified by Schondel, Schields, and Orel are similar to six needs identified by Clary, Snyder, and Ridge (1992). By involving themselves in volunteer work, volunteers may be hoping to satisfy personal needs:

1. *Social* reflects the influence of friends, family, or expectations of a social group.
2. *Values* allows the volunteer to act on deeply held beliefs about the importance of helping others, perhaps using the volunteer opportunity to advocate for a group or a cause that is important to the volunteer.
3. *Career* helps the volunteer explore job opportunities and introduces him or her to potential career contacts or particular career-related skills.
4. *Understanding* satisfies the desire to learn and understand the people whom one serves, the organization for which one volunteers, or oneself.
5. *Protective* provides relief or escape from negative feelings about oneself, loneliness, or guilt.
6. *Esteem* enhances a person's self-esteem by making the person feel needed and important.

These needs appear to be met in service learning programs.

Respondents in a national study of twenty-seven experiential education programs (ones integral to the general school curriculum but outside of the conventional classroom) for adolescents reported major gains in

- concern for others;
- ability to get things done and to work smoothly with others;
- development of realistic attitudes toward other people, such as the elderly, handicapped, or government officials;
- self-motivation to learn, participate, and achieve;
- self-concept;
- responsibility to the group or class;
- openness to new experiences;
- sense of usefulness in relation to the community;
- problem solving; and
- being assertive and independent. (Conrad and Hedin, 1982)

Additional studies have focused on the development of caring attitudes and behavior and indices of social development (Hamilton and Fenzel, 1988; Hart and Fegley, 1995). Others have begun to study the processes of change that the individual adolescent experiences during this maturation process (Pyle, 1981; Yates and Youniss, 1996). Pyle looks at cross-cultural service learning as a means of providing a developmental opportunity for experiencing the incongruity or dissonance necessary for an individual to relate her or his own opinions to other unfamiliar data. Drawing on the educational theory of Perry (1979), Pyle (1981) agreed that as students are faced with unfamiliar situations, they are taking in material from many sources at once and making decisions about what to do with that information. If this process happens in a situation where the student feels overwhelmed, the student may seek to escape from the fear and pressure. If, however, the student feels challenged and supported to face the risks in a new ego-threatening situation, identity development may be accelerated. Of the thirteen variables used by Pyle (1981) to measure student development, after a three-week service trip to Jamaica, significant gains were found in four variables relating particularly to development of mature life plans, autonomy, and interdependence. Pyle (1981) defines interdependence as "the realization by one that loving and being loved are complementary and that there is a direct relationship between one's own behavior and community welfare in general." Pyle (1981) saw the group as being a crucial part of this developmental process: "Experiencing together a new and different environment and having the emotional experience of working together as a team toward certain goals were essential ingredients of the program." A preliminary investigation by Burrus (1997) supports the significance of the group connections through a service experience by continued networking among group members six to twelve years later.

Yates and Youniss (1996) looked specifically at the effects of community service on adolescents and their identity development. With their focus not only on individual behavior, but also on that individual in relation to community welfare in general, Yates and Youniss (1996) use a tool for measuring these relationships in the context of transcendent narrative which links everyday reality to something beyond that reality. These narratives "acknowledge the present moment within a historical framework that acknowledges the past and anticipates the future . . . the here and now of immediate experience is incorporated within an interpretive process that allows transcendent meaning" (Yates and Youniss, 1996, p. 276).

Although the significance of peer group support is identified by Pyle (1981) and Burrus (1997), and the process of transcendence development and individual identity through service experiences is discussed by Yates and Youniss (1996), there has been no investigation of the effect of the group process on individual development during service learning experiences. Social group work literature contains a plethora of conceptual material on individual change through small group process (see, for example, Glasser, Sarri, and Vinter, 1974; Garvin and Seabury, 1997; Brown, 1991; Levine, 1967). The conceptual frameworks and studies which describe individual change through the group process, on many levels and within many contexts, suggest that group work intervention before, during, and after a service learning experience could facilitate individual identity development.

THE FIELD PLACEMENT

For the past three years, two faculty members of Marywood's Graduate School of Social Work have been conducting research on the various effects of service experiences on students' career choices and subsequent volunteer service. Preliminary results of these studies show that community service can be a powerful life-changing event in a student's college career and this individual effect is enhanced by participation in a mutual aid group in both preparation and provision of service (Gumpert and Twiss, 1995). As a result of these findings, a cooperative project was launched between the School of Social Work and Campus Ministry. Through this new arrangement, graduate social work students can elect a group work and/or administrative second year placement through Campus Ministry's Collegiate Volunteers, working with the Spring Break Service Trips. A faculty member with extensive experience in social group work and administration provides field instruction. Two of the authors were the first students in this placement and the third author is the field instructor. MSW students have been required to complete the elective course on social work practice with groups prior to or during their practicum at this site.

The expectations of undergraduate students participating in Spring Break Service Trips significantly shifted from Marywood's previous service trip learning expectations, which involved individual and academic preparation as well as competitive individual fund-raising. Group check-in sessions usually focused on fund-raising/financial matters, team-building exercises, readings on Appalachia and concerns about the trip itself, keeping a journal, and, finally, the reflection papers students were required to write based on their experiences. The new project emphasized the group process. The groups, formed by the social work students, were expected to meet for two hours each week, for ten weeks prior to spring break. They were to work together as a group in order to prepare for the trip financially, intellectually, and emotionally. Initial fund-raising to support the Spring Break Service Trips was used as a vehicle to facilitate group development. Social work students accompanied the undergraduates on the trip, and while in Appalachia, they met with the groups daily for approximately one hour to process the experiences of the day. Group meetings also continued for at least two sessions after their return for further reflection on the entire experience.

The graduate students developed a new application form and an interview guide. In their applications and interviews undergraduate students expressed all of the personal needs of volunteers identified by Clary, Snyder, and Ridge (1992) (social, values, career, understanding, protective, and esteem). These interviews, new to the application process, consisted of questions that generated information that was used to determine acceptance for the Spring Break Service Trips as well as decisions about group formation. When forming the different groups of students, specific factors were kept in mind. In order to assure group vitality, heterogeneity was built around the year of study, national origin (a mix of U.S. and international students), communication skills, previous service trip experiences, and typical roles each student adopted in a group setting. To facilitate group support, students who wished to travel together were placed in the same group. In coherence with the significance of the specific role or activity of the volunteers (Sundeen, 1992), whenever possible, undergraduate students were placed at sites that they had indicated as being their first choice.

Outside factors forced the formation of smaller than desirable groups (trip sites had limited places available due in part to the early scheduling of Marywood's spring break). Both groups (initially five members) lost one member during the beginning phase. All of the participants were female and ranged from freshmen to seniors with majors in a wide variety of disciplines and programs. The groups consisted of U.S. citizens and international students. Scheduling of meetings was surprisingly difficult because of the busy class, work, and extracurricular activities of the group members. This dynamic was used by both graduate students to develop negotiation and decision-making processes within the groups.

Power and control issues between the groups and the graduate students occurred in relation to the expectations of students going on these trips. Although the verbal conflict focused on the obligatory participation in the weekly two-hour meetings prior to the trip, it probably reflected resistance to change and the expectation of greater engagement of the undergraduate students. However, this issue was resolved during the Spring Break Service Trip.

Various program activities were used during the beginning phase of the group process. Group-oriented fund-raising activities consisted of selling raffle tickets at a university jazz brunch and a neighborhood convenience store and organizing and operating a flea market held at the university. Because several of the young women were concerned that they would be expected to cook for themselves on the trip, one group made dinner for the other group as a trial run. In anticipation of the trip site, a shelter for abused women, both groups invited a graduate social work student completing her practicum at the local women's shelter to their meetings to explore issues concerning spouse abuse. One graduate student brought in a tape of an interview with a regional author as an introduction to Southern dialects and culture. In another group, one of the members, spurred by questions about the terrain, looked for library resources about the Appalachian countryside.

Activities while on the trip consisted of cleaning up the grounds, clearing a drainage ditch in anticipation of spring rain, sorting clothes and assisting customers in the thrift shop, as well as helping with the cooking and cleaning for the residents and workers at the shelter. A member of the shelter's board, a local historian, spoke to the groups about the history and culture of the region. At his suggestion, the students attended a local high school basketball game and toured the region, observing the effects of poverty on small rural towns.

An unanticipated dynamic was the merging of the two groups once they reached the trip site. Because Marywood's spring break was earlier than many other schools, these two groups of four were the only students at the site for the week. They had spent time together at the dinner that one group prepared for the other and had traveled together in the same van to Appalachia. When they arrived, suddenly the students became conscious of the close ties with their own groups and the apparent exclusion of the other group. Wanting to do something about this exclusion, both groups independently decided to reach out to the other and, from the second day, began to function as one group. The small size of the initial groups may have contributed to this dynamic. The cohesion deepened in the middle of the week when during a picnic each of the students shared how she had come to this point in her life. The theme of this discussion was the recognition that apparently insignificant events could lead to major shifts in direction and new experiences. This cohesion was strengthened through decision making around a crisis when the van broke down and had to be repaired before it would be safe to make the return trip. This meant that everyone would arrive home one day later than anticipated.

EFFECTS OF THE GROUP WORK INTERVENTION

Observations of the graduate students and evaluations from the undergraduates indicate that, as Pyle (1981) noted, the group was a significant support system to students as they engaged in these new experiences. The group members' evaluation of the experience indicated that group ties were strong and helpful. Members were forced to think more about their experience than they had anticipated and they gained greater insight into the problem of violence and abuse. Graduate students observed that when students felt overwhelmed, other group members provided the support that was needed to help everyone face the risks in unfamiliar situations. During the trip, group roles were shared among members, cohesion was strong, and a new level of intimacy was reached. Relationships among group members have extended beyond these Spring Break Service Trips. Lasting friendships continue and many of the members are engaged in further service work.

As mentioned earlier, Yates and Youniss (1996) focused their study on the process through which community service stimulates identity development in adolescents. These authors use as their theoretical framework Erikson's elaboration of identity found in the prologue of *Identity, Youth and Crisis* (1968). In this volume, Erikson stressed the sociohistorical component of identity, pointing to the significance of the surrounding environment of which the youth is a part, on the process of identity formation. Yates and Youniss (1996) point out, "Erikson proposed that youths need to identify with values that have transcendence, that is, that supersede family and self and have historical continuity commanding respect from others who have lived and will live after them" (p. 273). These researchers suggest that institutions such as schools, churches, and other community organizations are the value-bearing institutions that present alternative values related to transcendence. These organizations connect youths to their communities by fostering relationships with adults, peers, and family and by promoting a prosocial set of norms that may continue into adulthood. This conceptual framework was of particular interest because it suggests the mechanism for having long-term effects on these students' behavior as they move into adulthood.

The recognized significance of peers in adolescent identity development would suggest that integrating this exposure through a group experience with peers would have a significant impact. The opportunity exists to share and discuss perspectives, values, and reactions, and to develop identity with a cohort of peers who share similar values in relation to past and future generations.

Using this theoretical backdrop, Yates and Youniss (1996) developed a tool that operationalized transcendence into three levels, moving from "little" to "big" and from "concrete" to "abstract":

> *Level 1:* Students see "other" as a person rather than as a stereotype or view "other" as an ordinary person who could be anyone.
> *Level 2:* Students confront consciousness of everyday life or compare their fortune to "others'" lot.
> *Level 3:* Students reflect on justice and responsibility or theorize about changing specific social problems, society, or political processes. (pp. 276-277)

Yates and Youniss (1996) suggest that this schema may measure a developmental process; with repeated experience, transcendent ideas grow from the immediate and concrete to the more general and abstract.

A particular focus of this project was whether the purposeful group intervention in the service experience facilitated group members' movement through the levels of transcendence. Although a systematic study of the transcendence process with groups was not completed, evidence suggests that these young adults moved through levels of transcendence. Following are some group interactions that exemplify this development (see appendix).

Level 1. In her discussion of the Spring Break Service Trip the previous year, a member describes her surprise that the people she met in Appalachia did not fit her stereotype. Another student questions whether she would be able to relate normally to the people in Appalachia. The group member reassures her that they will be able to relate to the people they will be meeting. The group discussion moves into the first level of transcendence: recognizing "other" as an ordinary person.

Level 2. Students confronted their own consciousness of everyday life in comparison to another's lot in their discussion about times when they felt homeless. Each member shares her own experience and then the group generalizes, comparing their experiences to the homeless. This discussion appears to move to the second level of transcendence: comparing one's fate with that of the "other."

Level 3. One of the members compares her fortune to the people in Appalachia, assuming that they will receive good help because the site is Christian sponsored. Another group member confronts that assumption, saying that a shelter can be good without it being religiously sponsored. Another group member begins to question the connection between religion and "good" behavior. Group members begin to define what is "just" and "right." This appears to be a group discussion, that moves to the third transcendence level: reflecting on justice and responsibility.

The group experience of service trips offers further possibilities for identity development for young adults. Through the group interaction focused on the experience of the "other," transcendence is fostered, prosocial values are reinforced as emerging group values, and the generational place in social history is developed through interaction with peers who share experiences and hold similar values. Using Erikson's formulation, the small group is one of the surrounding systems of which the individual is a part and therefore has an impact on identity development.

The poem "Making a River," written by this group on their last night of the Spring Break Service Trip, probably best captures the essence of the group service experience about which this chapter is written.

To our new friends, from the group.

MAKING A RIVER

We were a long, long way from home, but we were not
    all alone.
We came with strangers, we came with friends.
It is as friends that our journey ends.
Work was easy, work was fun.
We did have time to spend in the sun.
We hiked a mountain and dug a ditch.
When we hit the pickers we began to itch.
There was our meal prep, clean up too, then time for
    what we wanted to do.
Our late night talks would knock you off your socks,
and our games of basketball were fun for all.
The people we met were really neat, actually, they were
    really sweet

with personalities no one can beat.
There was J, L, and D too,
C and B, old friends now, who once were new.
B, N, J, B . . . they liked to hang out and just let loose.
L is a special case whom we often referred to as "Ace."

Our time here was short, our memories are long here . . .
    listen to our theme song.
We're "Making a River" that will flow strong.
It's the river connecting our friendship bond.
"Association" Bulgarian game was played.
As a group we talked.
As a group we laughed.
As a group we worked.
That is how OUR time passed.
We learned so much from all of you, most of which was
    very new.
But what we learned the most from all this fun, is that as
    a team,
We can get anything done!

FUTURE DIRECTIONS

Although this discussion and observations of this experience, viewing it with hindsight, strongly suggest that the intervention of social group workers helped to strengthen, deepen, and solidify the meaning of the service trip for the undergraduate students, systematic study is necessary to verify this effect and further explore contributing factors. It appears that the group interaction facilitated movement through the levels of transcendence, but this process also needs further study. Another exploration of interest would be whether it is possible for groups to move through levels of transcendence or whether individual members can move through levels of transcendence through group interaction but be at different levels in relation to one another.

Comparisons with service experiences, which do not include a group experience facilitated by a professional social group worker, would also be of interest. Longitudinal studies to focus on the enduring effects could better answer questions related to the capacity of these interventions to effect a qualitative change in attitudes toward social justice in the long term.

This discussion definitely suggests service learning trips with adolescents and young adults as a new arena for the use of social group work. The social group worker's focus on group development, autonomy, decision making, and purposeful use of program media in relation to individual identity development, group exploration, and group learning provides the expertise needed to help each individual member fully incorporate the growth this experience offers. In addition, a professional social worker's knowledge about social problems, the helping process, and individual-environment interaction allows her or him to be a rich resource for the discussions of groups. This arena for practice moves social group work back to its historical roots at the same time that it endorses enhancement of social functioning as an appropriate area for group intervention.

APPENDIX:
LEVELS OF TRANSCENDENCE IDENTIFIED
IN GROUP INTERACTION

Level 1—Recognizing "Other" As an Ordinary Person

CINDY: [Describing her trip to Appalachia the year before] I was surprised to see how friendly they were. They were real open about their lives . . . more so than us.

ANN: So, you didn't feel like a phony being down there to help them?

CINDY: No, not at all. . . . They were real accepting of us.

ANN: I didn't want to patronize them like we were just going down there to observe them.

CINDY: Yeah, we're just there to be their friends, not like we're some benevolent person looking down to help them up.

WORKER: Was anything different in the way that they lived and the way we live in Pennsylvania?

CINDY: They live far apart. The houses were falling apart. They don't keep them up.

ANN: So, that's how they're poor.

Level 2—Comparing One's Fate with That of "Other"

EMILY: [In response to the worker's question about homelessness] I knew in the back of my mind that I would have a place to go when I had to switch host families, but it was very unnerving.

FAITH: I had a similar experience when I ran away from home when I was younger . . . but I always knew I could go home.

GLADYS: When I went camping with the Girl Scouts we'd put ourselves in the position of being homeless . . . but we always brought our own food and shelter.

FAITH: There are some things you could do to prepare . . . but not really.

GLADYS: That's why it's really important to know where to go for help and that there are people who care enough to provide places for people to be until they get things figured out.

EMILY: Life is so unpredictable sometimes . . . you really usually don't plan to be homeless. It's really impossible to know when you might find yourself in the same predicament.

FAITH: My goodness, we are a very philosophical group.

Level 3—Reflecting on Justice and Responsibility

ANN: I'm glad the shelter is Christian. That will only make the healing process better. I've had some difficult times in my life and God has helped me through them.

BETTY: I don't think you have to have the shelter be Christian for them to be healed better. You can have a good shelter without it being religious.

DOROTHY: Well, I'm agnostic and it's possible to have people who go to church and do bad things the rest of the week and there are people who don't go to church and do good things. The important thing is to do the right thing.

WORKER: What is the right thing?

DOROTHY: The right thing is not to lie.

BETH: The right thing for me is to respect other people even though their opinions are different.

REFERENCES

Addams, J. (1910). *Twenty Years at Hull House*. New York: Macmillan.

Briggs, A. and Macartney, A. (1984). *Toynbee Hall, the First Hundred Years*. London and Boston: Routledge and Kegan Paul Publishers.

Brown, L. (1991). *Groups for Growth and Change.* New York: Longman.

Burrus, S. (1997). Marywood College's Service Trips to Appalachia: Continued Impact. Unpublished Study. School of Social Work, Marywood College.

Clary, E., Snyder, M., and Ridge, R. (1992). Volunteers' motivations: A functional strategy for the recruitment, placement, and retention of volunteers. *Nonprofit Management and Leadership,* 2(4), 333-350.

Conrad, D. and Hedin, D. (1982). The impact of experiential education on adolescent development. *Child and Youth Services,* 4(3/4), 57-76.

Erikson, E. (1968). *Identity, Youth and Crisis.* New York: Norton and Company.

Garvin, C. and Seabury, B. (1997). *Interpersonal Practice in Social Work: Promoting Competence and Social Justice.* Boston: Allyn and Bacon.

Glasser, P., Sarri, R., and Vinter, R. (1974). *Individual Change Through Small Groups.* New York: Free Press.

Gumpert, J. and Twiss, P. (1995). Building Bridges, Building Housing: Technical Report on Marywood Service Trips to Appalachia. Unpublished Report. Marywood University, Scranton, Pennsylvania.

Hamilton, S. and Fenzel, L. (1988). The impact of volunteer experience on adolescent social development: Evidence of program effects. *Journal of Adolescent Research,* 3(1), 65-80.

Hart, D. and Fegley, S. (1995). Prosocial behaviour and caring in adolescence: Relations to self-understanding and social judgment. *Child Development,* 66, 1346-1359.

Levine, B. (1967). *Fundamentals of Group Treatment.* Northbrook, IL: Whitehall Company.

Marriott, M. (1996). Taking education beyond the classroom. *The New York Times* (Education Life Section), August 4, pp. 22, 25, 38-39, 40.

Niebuhr, G. (1996). Colleges setting moral compasses. *The New York Times* (Education Life Section), August 4, pp. 23-24, 31.

Perry, W.G. (1979). Education that empowers. *The Synergist,* 8, 4-9.

Pyle, K. (1981). International cross-cultural service learning: Impact on student development. *Journal of College Student Personnel,* 22(6), 509-514.

Schondel, C., Shields, G., and Orel, N. (1992). Development of an instrument to measure volunteer's motivation in work with people with AIDS. *Social Work in Health Care,* 17(2), 53-71.

Smith, D.H. (1994). Determinants of voluntary association participation and volunteering: A literature review. *Nonprofit and Voluntary Sector Quarterly,* 23(3), 243-263.

Sundeen, R. (1992). Differences in personal goals and attitudes among professionals. *Nonprofit and Voluntary Sector Quarterly,* 21(3), 271-291.

Yates, M. and Youniss, J. (1996). Community service and political-moral identity in adolescents. *Journal of Research on Adolescence,* 6(3), 271-284.

Chapter 7

The Use of Teleconferencing Focus Groups with Families Involved in Organ Donation: Dealing with Sensitive Topics

Sandra Regan

The focus group technique has substantial potential for providing information that is simultaneously relevant to sociological investigations and is difficult to obtain using other techniques (e.g., surveys, experiments, etc.). It offers the promise of providing definitions to the situation that would not otherwise be available to the researcher. In particular, the focus group can provide information on sensitive topics about which respondents are usually reticent to talk. To capitalise on this promise, the researcher needs to employ those interaction principles that will foster and encourage discussion about these sensitive topics (Zeller, 1993, p. 182).

This chapter is directed to group work practitioners and researchers who are considering using teleconferencing focus groups to deal with sensitive topics. It explores the use of time-limited teleconferencing focus groups with families who have been involved in organ donation. It concentrates on the preparation and the beginning stage of the focus group, for it is here that an environment for dealing with sensitive topics needs to be created. Once this has occurred, the group moves on to discussions that would occur in any focus group. The chapter emphasises what needs to be done in order for the focus group to arrive at this point.

WHY TELECONFERENCING FOCUS GROUPS?

Technology is having an impact on most types of research, and focus group interviewing is no exception. An increasingly com-

mon approach to reaching individuals who are dispersed geo-
graphically or otherwise difficult to reach is the use of a conference telephone call as a substitute for a face-to-face group meeting. Teleconferencing greatly expands the pool of potential
participants and adds considerable flexibility to the process of
scheduling an interview. (Stewart and Shamdasani, 1990, p. 60)

Teleconferencing focus groups were decided on in this instance
because prospective participants were small in number and spread
over a wide geographic area, making face-to-face groups impossible.
Due to the nature of organ donation, the families of organ donors are
never likely to form a natural group: access to one another is ordi-
narily impossible or extremely unlikely.

Teleconferencing focus groups also offered the potential of exploring the use of teleconferencing with this population. This was of particular significance as the purpose of the focus groups was to identify
needs and then consider how they could be addressed in teleconferencing group counselling. Follow-up support and counselling is
important for these families because they have suffered immense loss
and, as Douglass and Daly (1995) acknowledge, bereavement support after donation is an essential part of assisting the donor's family
in working through the grieving process.

As focus groups were conducted via teleconferencing, it is important to recognize the advantages and disadvantages of this means of
gathering information:

Focus group interviewing via teleconferencing may be the only
option for certain types of samples, but it is not without some
cost relative to more traditional groups. The lack of face-to-face
interaction often reduces the spontaneity of the group and eliminates the nonverbal communication that plays a key role in elic-
iting responses. Such nonverbal communication is often critical
for determining when further questioning or probing will be
useful, and is often an important source of interplay among
group members. Teleconferencing tends to reduce the intimacy
of the group as well, making group members less likely to share
more personal or sensitive information. Finally, the moderators'
role is made more difficult because it is harder to control the participants. Dominant participants are more difficult to quiet, and

less active participants are more difficult to recognize. (Stewart and Shamdasani, 1990, p. 60)

Some of Stewart and Shamdasani's comments need qualification, based on experiences with families of organ donors in the teleconferencing focus groups discussed in this chapter. Although the lack of face-to-face interaction initially reduced spontaneity, eventually it allowed people to express thoughts and feelings that would have been perhaps more difficult in a face-to-face group. When others' nonverbals cannot be seen, participants are more likely to concentrate on taking care of their own personal needs. The absence of nonverbals may work for the groups rather than against them.

In these groups, teleconferencing did not reduce intimacy as Stewart and Shamdasani (1990) suggest. Anonymity actually enhanced the intimacy. Anonymity in teleconferencing provides protection where people feel free to say things they would not necessarily say in a face-to-face group. Having the chance to share needs created an immediate sense of connection. The emotive nature of the sensitive topics enhanced the power of this bond.

To ensure that all participants had an opportunity to share their identified needs, at the begining of the session, each person was asked to share his or her particular needs. However, each individual was free to decide how much to contribute. If the group went on to interact with one another, the moderators did not interrupt. Moderators checked in with other members only when cross talk stopped. Participants had a great deal of respect for one another's pain and this created a willingness to share as well as a willingness to listen. All the above made the moderators' role easier and permitted everyone to participate.

Although Stewart and Shamdasani (1990) describe disadvantages associated with teleconferencing, they also recognize its potential: "Despite these limitations, teleconferencing has become an important tool for conducting focus groups among hard-to-reach respondents" (Stewart and Shamdasani, 1990, p. 60).

DEALING WITH SENSITIVE TOPICS

Teleconferencing focus groups provide the opportunity to explore sensitive topics. They can provide a sense of comfort and encourage information exchange. However, one also needs to consider a means to provide a safe environment that encourages participation.

For the purposes of this chapter, the organ donation process, including sudden loss, brain death, and the donation, must be understood. All happen within a limited time frame. "An association between sudden death, with its attendant grief and the destructive effect on individual and family stability, and organ donation when it occurs, is unavoidable" (Pearson et al., 1995, p. 93).

Many assume this automatic association and may need to address these sensitive topics together. However, this association does not negate their separateness and the different issues surrounding each individual. They are separate. Facing sudden loss and brain death precedes the organ donation. Yet, all three are linked in the bereavement process which occurs with sudden death and which continues as the reality of the loss sets in.

> Sudden death as a consequence of an acute severe brain injury is the essential and inevitable precursor to the donation of most solid organs. For most families of such patients, this is also the first occasion for any real association with brain death. There is no preparation for the onslaught of sudden death on the integrity of the family unit, none of the protection that might be conferred when death is expected, and usually, no educational basis for any insight into the horrifying idea of a destroyed brain within a seemingly living being. (Pearson et al., 1995, p. 88)

Every family of an organ donor has to deal with the concept of brain death. This is a very difficult concept as it forces people to rethink their ideas of what constitutes death. For most people, death is based on the idea that the heart and breathing stop. The brain dead organ donor is apparently alive. He or she has the appearance of breathing and the heart is still beating. The body is still warm.

It is only after brain death has been confirmed that families are approached regarding organ donation. If consent to organ donation is given, then support before, during, and after the organ donation is important. Whatever their decision, the family needs help in dealing with the circumstances surrounding the death.

A few additional comments on the families of organ donors are necessary. When considering families of organ donors, it is important to think of the individuals who constitute the family. The organ donation process may entail many family members. However, each individual family member will have his or her own needs and handle the bereavement process differently. There is no one way to deal with the bereavement process, and consideration must be given to physical and psychological factors, the relationship of the deceased person to the bereaved, the age of the deceased, circumstances of death, and the family support system.

In the focus groups to be presented, it is individual family members who participate, not the family as a whole. What can be done to ease the introduction of sensitive topics to these individuals in the focus groups?

Zeller (1993) has written about the use of focus groups for dealing with sensitive topics such as sexual decision making. Although the content to be considered by donor families is different from matters relating to sex, there are still some similarities in process:

> A focus group researcher can use a variety of tools for setting the agenda of a focus group on sensitive topics. This needs to be done without producing excessively socially desirable responses. These tools include the screener questionnaire, the introductory comments before the focus group session, and reactions to participants' comments during the focus group session. (Zeller, 1993, p. 167)

Zeller (1993) further refined these points into reactivity to the screener questionnaire, moderator self-disclosure in the introductory comments, and legitimisation of participant comments. These will be considered and expanded to include motivation of participants, credibility of moderator, self-disclosure of group members, and normalisation of emotions.

I shall now discuss reactivity to the screener questionnaire and how this contributed to the teleconferencing focus groups for families involved in organ donation.

REACTIVITY IN THE SCREENER QUESTIONNAIRE

"Reactivity refers to the phenomenon that the very process of measurement can induce change in the phenomenon itself" (Zeller, 1993, p. 168). Zeller (1993) argues that reactivity should be taken advantage of and used to help focus participants' thinking about the topic before the group begins. He views a screener questionnaire as one way of ensuring that this happens.

In 1995, a donor family survey was conducted by the Coordinator of Bereavement Services for the Next Step Programme of the New South Wales (NSW) Red Cross Blood Transfusion Service (BTS). The purpose of the survey was to evaluate and provide a better overall service to donor families. In retrospect, the survey could also be perceived as a screener questionnaire. A letter was sent to 104 families who had previously indicated a desire to be on a mailing list for the annual ecumenical service, to ascertain interest in participating in a survey. In NSW and Australian Capital Territory, the coordination of organ donation is facilitated via the NSW Red Cross BTS.

Of the 104 families contacted, fifty individual family members consented to participate in the survey. Forty returned completed questionnaires for a response rate of 80 percent. The survey included two major themes: (1) the experience of the family in the intensive care unit, their understanding of brain death, and the approach for organ donation; and (2) the follow-up they received, whether it was appropriate, helpful, and if not, what could have been useful. These could also be considered as screener questions, as the purpose of the focus group was to discuss identified needs in relation to these sensitive topics.

Issues that related to counselling services, particularly with regards to follow-up and contact with both rural and urban donor families were of concern. This was also evident in the research of Douglass and Daly (1995), who wrote of the lack of follow-up services provided to donor families in both rural and metropolitan areas of Queensland and who suggested that the donor families benefit from counselling in both the short and long term.

Respondents were asked if they would have been interested in joining a teleconferencing counselling group had it been available at the time of their bereavement. This became the most important screener question. Fifty-seven percent of the returned forty individual respondents answered positively. A letter was sent asking these respondents if they would like to participate in two focus group sessions, via teleconference, for a duration of one hour each.

The purpose of the focus group was explained, namely to identify the various needs the participants had during the organ donation and subsequent bereavement process as well as how these needs might be met in a teleconferencing group counselling service. This was further discussed when they were contacted and times arranged for the teleconference focus groups.

Of the respondents, twelve indicated a willingness to participate in a focus group and were available on the nights agreed to for the teleconferences. At a later date, one other individual agreed to participate. The thirteen participants were divided into two groups primarily based on time availability. The experience of organ donation ranged from as recently as eighteen months to as far back as six years.

As they were aware ahead of time that they would be asked about their own experiences and needs during the organ donation process, they were able to rethink the actual organ donation process as well as their needs. This had positive as well as negative aspects. It did help them identify needs. However, to do this, they revisited sad memories and faced unresolved grief. This was not an easy task for participants. Willingness to do so indicated a high degree of commitment and motivation. The moderators needed to be aware and responsive to the painful memories that could be evoked.

Each focus group included two one-hour sessions, one week apart. This allowed participants to think between sessions about what other group members had said. The ability to talk to other family members (as organ donation is a family experience) between sessions also added to the quality of the information shared. The second session offered an opportunity to revisit identified needs and ideas from the previous week and add new ones. As a final additional verification, a questionnaire was sent out one week after the second session, giving members the opportunity to identify any needs they wanted considered that had not previously been mentioned.

> The principle of reactivity suggests that the asking of such sensitive questions will alert the participants to those topics. While such awareness might threaten the validity of a survey or experiment, it is here argued that it enhances the value of the participants' comments in the focus group. This enhancement occurs because the time and attention that the participant devotes to the focus group is not only the 2 hours in the discussion but also the days or weeks before the focus group during which the participant is mulling over the issues raised reactively in the screener questionnaire. Participants are going to mull over what they say

before they say it. This issue is whether they have the opportunity to mull it over for minutes or days. (Zeller, 1993, p. 169)

The donor family survey inquired about needs in general and not about how they could be linked to teleconferencing group counselling. The quality of information obtained from the screener questionnaire was different from the teleconferencing focus groups. The screener questionnaire gained individual information while the teleconferencing focus groups gained individual information as well as group interactional information within clearly defined boundaries.

Reactivity occurred with the screener questionnaire. Whether this is perceived as positive or negative is open to debate. However, as a moderator, I believe the positives it offered to the groups assisted in a quick transition to sensitive topics. Now that we have an understanding of reactivity, the incentive/motivation of participants needs to be explored.

MOTIVATION OF THE PARTICIPANTS

Focus groups are a time-consuming activity for participants. Taking two or more hours out of one's life to talk to a group of strangers is not likely to be viewed as an appealing prospect, particularly if one has worked all day. There are a variety of incentives that may be used to encourage participation, and most focus group participants are provided monetary and other incentives. (Stewart and Shamdasani, 1990, p. 55)

Stewart and Shamdasani (1990) use the word "incentives," which links focus groups to market research, where monetary or in kind (e.g., travel) incentives are prevalent. For the focus groups under discussion, the term "motivation," which focuses more on the need or desire that causes a person to participate, seems to be a more appropriate term to capture the underlying dimensions attached to participation. The term "motivation" can also be used in a similar fashion when it relates to reasons that bring people to volunteer. Clary, Snyder, and Ridge (1992, cited in Dunn, 1995) claim that, in lieu of a tangible reward, each person who volunteers does so in an attempt to satisfy some sort of personal need.

Individual differences existed in motivation for member participation in the teleconferencing focus groups. However, the motivation most frequently acknowledged by participants was the desire to contribute towards defining and creating a new service that would help future families going through the organ donation process.

Other motives, such as the following, became apparent during the focus group experiences:

- A part of participants' way of going through the bereavement process. It helped consolidate some of their ideas and allowed them to retell their stories. It offered an opportunity to help others and the possibility of sharing with those in similar circumstances. It helped them regain some control over their own situations by being proactive rather than reactive.
- If participants had experienced something they felt was inappropriately handled in the organ donation process, they could inform others to ensure it did not happen again. It offered them the opportunity to be heard and acknowledged.
- Participants were able to talk about the deceased person with unconditional support and acceptance from others outside their family, with people who had experienced similar situations and therefore understand what it is really like. They could be themselves and did not need to cover up or protect others. No one was trying to stop them or put time limits on their bereavement.
- They saw participation as a way of helping the Red Cross to speed up the process of providing additional services.

As Stewart and Shamdasani (1990) note, "Incentives should be selected that have universal value to the participants, what may be valuable to one person may have little value to other" (1990, pp. 55-56). In the case of families of organ donors, the overriding motivation seemed to be helping others.

MODERATORS' SELF-DISCLOSURE AND CREDIBILITY

The self-disclosure and credibility of moderators contribute to a climate of trust and facilitate further self-disclosures. Zeller (1993) identifies moderator self-disclosure as a tool that could be used to increase the range of acceptable self-disclosure in focus groups. When working with families involved in the organ donation process, another important tool, linked to self-disclosure, is the establishment of the practitioners' credibility in relation to sensitive topics.

As these focus groups were conducted via teleconferencing, it was particularly important for moderators to recognize that the groups would be connected suddenly, with no time for gradual introductions prior to the group. The role call of members was handled by the telephone operator. The welcome needed to engage the participants immediately. First names were used because members could not see each other and it was important to identify who was speaking. Some comments about teleconferencing were provided, as for most participants it was a new way of connecting with others. The moderators' self-disclosure followed thereafter.

The coordinator of bereavement services, the donor coordinator, and the author served as moderators for the focus groups. It was decided to have comoderators due to the sensitive nature of topics under discussion and the different knowledge and skills each could bring to the group.

Both bereavement and donor coordinators had had previous contact with some of the group members. Rather than working against the group this worked to their advantage because it helped establish early credibility and provided some initial connections. However, the group very quickly moved beyond individual connection to group connections and everyone participated actively. Although moderators had counselling skills, it was made clear from the outset that this group was not for counselling but for needs assessment. Indeed, awareness of moderators' counselling skills seemed to increase feelings of security.

The role of the moderators was to establish the normalcy of the topic under discussion at the start of the focus group. This was enabled by self-disclosure and credibility. By this means moderators, within the first fifteen minutes, established rapport and connected the group around sensitive topics.

Moderators were introduced in terms of agency base, previous experience in bereavement counselling, involvement in the organ donation process, and skills in group work and teleconferencing. Self-disclosure in relation to work, not personal information, was used to establish the moderators' credibility. Their role was also explained as keeping the group on track and making sure everyone had an opportunity to participate.

It was important for moderators' comments about organ donation to be more detailed than would normally be accepted outside the group to encourage participants' self-disclosure. As the focus groups were dealing with sudden loss, brain death, and organ donation, moderators needed to be comfortable themselves discussing these topics. They needed to connect with but not take over the group. Moderators served as experts for the focus group process and participants were experts when it came to the content, for example with regard to their needs. The moderators were required to establish a level of expertise on sensitive topics and create a sense that it was safe to discuss them. The safety factor was the priority, for the more secure participants felt, the more they were likely to self-disclose.

In our society, sensitive topics are not usually discussed openly. A limit to the number of people with whom one can talk comfortably about these subjects exists, and one's own degree of comfort and ability to discuss them also comes into play.

> The reality of the loss comes and goes until it is gradually accepted as a fact. By that time, however, those who were initially supportive may no longer want to hear about the loss, expecting the bereaved person to be over their grief. Many people are intolerant of others' grief because it is a reminder that the same tragedy could occur in their own lives. (Cerney, 1993, p. 35)

This is the reaction many people have to death. Very few people, however, have any knowledge of brain death and organ donation. Few can identify meaningfully with the experience. When wanting to discuss brain death and organ donation, the number of people families may communicate with may be even more limited than in the case of death.

Moderators had to work quickly to ensure that societal norms did not carry over to the group. Thus, from the start, a new norm of self-disclosure around sudden loss, brain death, and organ donation needed to be created. What could be seen as excessive self-disclosure outside the group became the norm within this group. This high level of self-disclosure enhanced the degree of intimacy.

[P]articipants must be willing to say things in the focus group that are very unacceptable and clearly excessive disclosure in ordinary conversation if the endeavour is going to explore successfully sensitive topics. The moderator's goal is clear. The moderator must either change the definition of appropriate self-disclosure or fail to explore fully the sensitive topic; both cannot be simultaneously accomplished within one interaction setting. (Zeller, 1993, p. 178, emphasis in original)

To facilitate changing norms brought from outside the group, moderators clearly identified the purpose of the group before the session, incorporated reactivity from the prior donor family survey and identified various motivations for participating in the focus group. Members were also reminded that their self-disclosure enhanced this process.

GROUP MEMBERS' SELF-DISCLOSURE

After the moderators were introduced to the members, introduction of the members took place. By this time, on an intellectual level, the sensitive topics had been introduced by the moderators and a willingness to discuss them was demonstrated. It must be kept in mind that the only people who can actually change the norm concerning sensitive topics of the group are the members themselves. They could choose to discard an old norm and embrace a new one or maintain the status quo. Given all the prior work in establishing the focus of the group, participants were ready to discuss sudden loss, brain death, and organ donation.

Members were asked to introduce themselves by sharing a little about who they were, who had died, under which circumstances, and when. It is important to recognise just how difficult this was for the participants, as it is clearly distressing to revisit past pain and disturbing memories. However, this did not stop members from participating. After each speaker, the group gained strength by acknowledging commonalities.

The first introduction was the most difficult but after that everybody became more at ease in their contributions. Some hesitancy still existed, but with each successive introduction one could almost feel a sigh of relief that the group was actually going to engage in the business at hand and whatever was said would be accepted. In sharing their experiences, group members experienced instant connection. There was respect for the sharing, and a recognition of a need to talk to others who really understood what it was like to be a family, from a family perspective, involved in the organ donation process. In retrospect, they were perhaps more ready for a deeper level of sharing than originally expected by moderators. After all, it was their issue and they were experts in their own experience. Unitedly, the members decided upon what was appropriate, thus sustaining the new group norm.

As members were making their introductions, euphemisms were used to refer to sudden unexpected death, for example, "sudden loss," "passed away," "passed on," yet all members were explicit in the use of the term "brain death." Even though there were different levels of understanding about brain death, the term still created a commonality of language in the group that the word "death" alone did not convey. The use of the term "brain death" helped to connect the group.

This introduction allowed the members to talk about themselves as well as the deceased person. They were asked to share whatever they felt ready to at that point. Had the participants been uncomfortable with the new norm, introductions could have been very superficial. However, the opposite occurred and members immediately provided detailed information about their experiences.

NORMALISATION OF EMOTIONS

Once the norm of increased self-disclosure regarding sensitive topics was set, the emotional component of establishing new norms needed to be acknowledged. After facilitating introductions, the difficulties of the process for some were recognized and, at this point, the normalisation of emotions became the task of moderators. "It is sometimes difficult to consider, even in the abstract, the possibility of donating one's own organs, those of loved ones, and especially those of one's children" (Cerney, 1993, p. 36). For these group members, organ donation was no longer an abstraction. It had happened to them in reality with all the intense emotions attached. These emotions needed to be normalised.

Although teleconferencing focus groups were established to gain information, it is important to be aware of the other aspects of these groups. To obtain information, some uncomfortable emotions had to be accepted as part of the process. If at times members felt tearful or upset, this was acknowledged, understood, and accepted. The importance of this work together and the role teleconferencing group counselling could play in the future to help deal with these kinds of emotions and underlying needs was reflected in the intensity of work in the focus groups.

Although his comments are not specifically directed to dealing with strong emotions, Zeller (1993) recognizes the importance of conveying to participants that, should they not feel ready to speak, they are free to pass their turn. Because the organ donor groups were dealing with such strong emotions, it was essential for this point to be openly acknowledged.

Sometimes members needed simply to "sit with" an emotion or a thought for a short period. While that was acceptable, due to the lack of visual contact, a moderator might briefly check in with the member to ensure that all was well. Again, this provided a sense of safety in the group and helped to normalise the emotional components.

LEGITIMISATION OF PARTICIPANTS' COMMENTS

During the introduction, most of the communication was directed towards the moderator. However, one could tell if connections between members were being made by background noises, e.g., "um," "ah." If the next person linked their introduction to what a previous person said, a connection was clearly made. After the group members introduced themselves, the reasons for the establishment of focus groups were reiterated, thus reinforcing legitimation.

> Concerning legitimisation, moderators need to provide enough legitimation to ensure that the range of comments from socially desirable to socially undesirable are aired but not provide so much legitimation for one position that those holding other positions feel that their comments would not be well received. (Zeller, 1993, p. 183)

To facilitate this process, guidelines were provided. It was made clear that the group was to explore identified needs, not to make decisions. Members needed to share as many of their identified needs and ideas as possible. It was important to suspend judgement on what others said. They were asked to share needs, but not to look at them in relation to what they thought was the most important need, whether a need was realistic or unrealistic in terms of being met, or whether they felt more or less strongly about a particular need. A whole range of needs had to be canvassed. They were aware the two sessions were clearly divided. The first session focussed on needs identification; the second revisited identified needs, added new ones, and then began to consider the needs as they might relate to teleconferencing group counselling.

BUILDING ON PREPARATION
AND BEGINNING THE FOCUS GROUP

This chapter has discussed the preparation and beginning stage of two time-limited teleconferencing focus groups for families who have been involved in the organ donation process. What happened prior to the group as well as what happened in the first fifteen or twenty minutes of the first one-hour session sets the stage for the rest of the group. This time needed to be used wisely, as only forty minutes were left in the first session for discussion.

In the organ donor groups, the sessions were taped with the permission of all of the participants. Recording was essential to preserve all of the participants' ideas and to assist the moderators in preparing for the next session. Due to the demanding concentration level required in teleconferencing, content as well as process items could be easily missed had the moderators only used their notes. Taping also allowed moderators more time to deal with the emotional component. Moderators made some notes during the teleconference simply to keep track of participation frequency.

In the focus group discussion, the most commonly identified needs were dealing with others (e.g., doctors, nurses, etc.) in times of stress, the need for information during and after the organ donation process, understanding brain death, and acknowledgement from organ recipients. There were many variations within each of these needs that offer the potential for exploration within teleconferencing group counselling.

CONCLUSION

The special and sharing people who participated in these teleconferencing focus groups must be acknowledged. They gave of themselves willingly and this was evident throughout the group sessions. The challenge for participants to revisit the organ donation experience and deal with the continuing bereavement process should not be minimised. These focus groups reinforced the need for counselling services and their outcome will assist in setting up a teleconferencing group counselling service within the Next Step Programme of the NSW Red Cross BTS. "Not everyone can use professional help in the aftermath of tragedy. But if the counselling service were available over a 2-year period, help would be available when needed later to prevent or interrupt maladaptive adjustment behavior" (Cerney, 1993, p. 35).

This chapter aimed to demonstrate the value of teleconferencing focus groups in dealing with sensitive topics. To illustrate, it used teleconferencing focus groups with families of organ donors who are dealing with sudden loss, brain death, and organ donation. It highlighted the process of discussing sensitive topics through elaboration of reactivity to a screener questionnaire, motivations of participants, moderators' credibility, group members' self-disclosure, normalisation of emotions, and legitimisation of participants' comments. If all of these components are handled appropriately, then the ensuing discussion should be active and informative. This was so with the teleconferencing focus groups for families involved in organ donation, families who would otherwise be denied the opportunity of sharing their identified needs within a supportive group environment.

REFERENCES

Cerney, M.S. (1993). Solving the organ donor shortage by meeting the bereaved family's needs. *Critical Care Nurse*, February, 32-36.

Clary, F., Snyder, M., and Ridge, R. (1992). Volunteers' motivations: A functional strategy for the recruitment, placement, and retention of volunteers. *Nonprofit Management and Leadership*, 2(4), 333-350.

Douglass, G.E. and Daly, M. (1995). Donor families' experience of organ donation. *Anaesthesia and Intensive Care*, 23(1).

Dunn, D. (1995). Motivations for giving: Consent for the donation of organs and tissues. *Journal of Transplant Coordination*, 5, 2-8.

Morgan, D.L. (1988). *Focus Groups As Qualitative Research,* Volume 16. London: Sage Publications.

Pearson, I.Y., Bazeley, T., Spencer-Plane, Chapman, J.R., and Robertson, P. (1995). A survey of families of brain dead patients: Their experiences, attitudes to organ donation and transplantation. *Anaesthesia and Intensive Care,* 23(1), 88-95.

Pittman, S. (1985). Alpha and omega: The grief of the heart donor family. *The Medical Journal of Australia,* 143, 568-570.

Stewart, D.W. and Shamdasani, P.N. (1990). *Focus Groups: Theory and Practice, Applied Social Research Methods Series,* Volume 20. London: Sage Publications.

Zeller, R.A. (1993). Focus group research on sensitive topics: Setting the agenda without setting the agenda. In Morgan, D. (Ed.), *Successful Focus Groups: Advancing the State of the Art* (pp. 167-183). London: Sage Publications.

Chapter 8

Using Groups for Research and Action: The Asian Mothers' Support Project

Lorraine Gutiérrez
Izumi Sakamoto
Tom Morson

The University of Michigan is one of the most international universities in the United States. In 1996, one in twelve of all enrolled students came from another country. On the graduate level, the proportion of international students doubled to more than one in six, with as many as 40 percent in the engineering school. Twenty-five percent of graduate student instructors are international; three out of five Rackham Distinguished Dissertation Awards were given to international students in 1997; and the university hosts a number of visiting international scholars and their families. Married international students and scholars bring their families; half of the campus family housing apartment units are leased to international students and scholars (3,500 or more residents), the majority of whom are from Asia. The international populations are an integral part of the academic and intellectual life of the university.

Although the contributions made by international families to campus and community life are recognized, the needs of this population are often ignored. Few programs exist to address the stresses experienced by individuals and families who have moved, often away from established families and friends, to a new life in an unfamiliar culture.

This project is supported by funding from the Society for the Psychological Study of Social Issues; the Japanese Business Society of Detroit; and Counseling and Psychological Services, the School of Social Work, and the Department of Psychology at the University of Michigan.

This can be especially stressful for the partners and other family members of students who do not have the structure created by school and jobs and who may not have fluent English language ability. Often, these family members are not eligible for university support services such as counseling and information services.

This chapter presents program information and data from an action research project developed to address the experiences of international families at the University of Michigan. This program involves students, university staff, faculty, and international students in a collaborative group-based project. The resulting mix of interests and expertise has made for a productive synergy. This collaboration brings together the worlds of the researcher and the practitioner and of faculty, staff, and students, offering each participant an expanded awareness and a learning opportunity. It also provides much needed assessment, evaluation, and service offerings for international student families. Our overall approach has been based on the *empowerment praxis* —multiple cycles of research, action, and reflection in the creation and implementation of programs. This program can be particularly relevant to group work practitioners because of the way in which the groups were used for a variety of objectives—planning, research, services, and action.

THE NORTH CAMPUS OUTREACH PROJECT

All of the supportive services and activities available for students and their families have lacked the ability to address the needs of international students and families, who represent half of the residents living in family housing (University of Michigan Housing International Students Committee, 1991). Although Ann Arbor is more international than many other cities its size in the Midwest, it does not have established communities of immigrants from different countries. International spouses, more often women than men, are "transplanted" and often do not have any formal connections to the university. They may have a much harder time adjusting to the new context than their partners who came to study at the university (University of Michigan International Center, 1996). When Counseling and Psychological Services conducted a survey in the early 1990s, many international students identified the need for services to their families and children regarding initial orientation, cultural adjustment, and parenting support.

Several other leading research universities (Institute of International Education, 1995; Schwartz and Kahne, 1993) provide programs for spouses in varied capacities with various programs located in the International Center (e.g., Stanford), in the Medical Center (e.g., MIT), and some in the self-help organizations (e.g., University of Washington). Very few programs have been developed to address the experiences of international families. During the 1980s, the university's Center for the Education of Women offered an internship program for international spouses interested in maintaining or increasing their work experience. The International Center also offered a series of workshops for international spouses focusing mainly on the issues related to job searching. Although these programs have been well received, they do not speak to many international spouses who experience barriers to work or even attending workshops due to nonworking visa status, limited English fluency, and lack of child care.

In response to these needs, Counseling and Psychological Services (CAPS), the International Center (IC), Family Housing (FH), the Sexual Assault and Prevention Center (SAPAC), and all offices of the Division of Student Affairs (DSA) at the University of Michigan, have been working collaboratively to meet the myriad needs of international students. Since 1993, an outreach office of CAPS, supported by FH, has existed near family housing to ease access for students residing there. In 1996, the IC also opened an office within the same vicinity.

Since implementing these programs, we have observed that those most often requesting services are the *spouses* of students. Our work with international families has often seemed to be in response to an extreme emergency. We were aware of the various obstacles related to making a successful transition into a new environment with different cultural expectations. Over the years, programs have been offered to address such concerns, but language and cultural barriers kept many of these families from participating. We felt stymied in our efforts to reach them. As they were "housebound" primary caregivers of children, with limited English fluency, lack of a work visa, and no formal university connection, the task seemed formidable.

The North Campus Outreach Project (NCOP) was initiated in the summer of 1996 to provide services for spouses and families of international Asian families living in family housing. The main goals of NCOP are to reach out and develop culturally sensitive services for this population in order to assist them in establishing, strengthening, and maintaining social support for one another and to help them cope with the transitional nature of cross-cultural stress. Ongoing assessments serve as the basis for providing services, and most of the services and research are conducted in various Asian languages to better reach those with limited English language ability.

International families have unique assets and needs that may not be accommodated by regular service providers due to cultural differences. Thus, this collaborative project included a team of scholars, community residents, and service providers who were involved in implementing services that attempted to meet the needs and draw upon the strengths of this unique population. NCOP received partial funding from the university's Counseling and Psychological Services, the Family Housing Office, Rackham School of Graduate Studies, Department of Psychology and School of Social Work, as well as the Japanese Business Society of Detroit and the Society for the Psychological Study of Social Issues.

A PROGRAM AND A PROCESS FOR CHANGE

NCOP was designed as an action research project based on methods for multicultural community development. A multicultural community development perspective involves a practice that recognizes and values the experiences and contributions of different social groups within the community while working to bring those groups together. It is built upon a pluralistic foundation but goes beyond pluralism by recognizing and working to eliminate social injustices and oppression based on group membership (Gutiérrez et al., 1996). This perspective recognizes and builds upon ways the capable community members have worked toward improving their living and community conditions. Working with and building upon community resources and institutions is an important means for utilizing and identifying community strengths while institutionalizing and building leadership and structures (Delgado and Humm-Delgado, 1982).

Action research methods were used to identify and understand community needs, strengths, and resources. Action research refers to research methods that are focused on developing knowledge that can be utilized readily (Brown, 1994). It was recognized that due to the closed and often transient nature of this community little empirical information regarding this group was available. Therefore, focus groups, program evaluations, and periodic surveys were conducted to learn more about the community and the degree to which programs were meeting the community's identified needs.

Focus Groups

Focus groups for Asian women were conducted in the summer of 1996 to explore the needs of international families. These focus groups were held in four different languages (Japanese, Korean, Mandarin, and English) at a community center located on North Campus. Child care and a continental breakfast were provided. Participants were recruited to the groups at community outreach presentations and through fliers taped to bus shelters and garbage bins. All recruitment materials were written in the targeted languages.

Female graduate students and a faculty member fluent in the specific languages conducted the focus groups. Facilitators followed an interview protocol developed to elicit residents' experiences in different areas of their lives. These areas included cultural adjustment, child rearing, couple relationships, and sources of social support. Focus group facilitators were trained to use techniques that encourage open communication and discussion around these topics.

The focus groups were well received by the participants. Twenty-two women and twenty children attended the groups. The majority of the women were Japanese (seven) or Korean (six) with Taiwanese, Chinese, Singaporean, and Vietnamese composing the remainder of the group. The average age was 32.47 (range twenty-six to thirty-eight); the average number of children was 1.4 (range one to three). The majority of children were preschool age, with a range of four months to nine years. The average participant had been in the United States for 2.15 years; however the majority had been in this country for less than two years.

These focus groups provided us with information regarding the needs and resources required by Asian spouses living on North Campus. These needs include the absence of child care (which inhibited broader community participation), the lack of information on health care and child abuse laws, the inaccessibility of services, life in general in Ann Arbor, and finally cultural and linguistic differences. Very few resources other than their spouses or neighbors were identified. Indeed, few women were aware of the scope and nature of programs and services available to them. Data collected from these groups enhanced our understanding of the nature of this community. Issues that were identified include the following.

Isolation Resulting from Cultural and Language Differences

The isolation experienced by many spouses of international students at the university has both cultural and structural causes. Language and cultural differences may isolate these women from the larger university community and may make it difficult for the university to provide services to these families. Their roles as spouses and primary caregivers for children can make it all the harder for them to break out of this isolation.

The stress experienced by sojourners resulting from difficulties adjusting to a new culture and lack of social support has been pointed out in cross-cultural education and counseling psychology literature (Pederson, 1995; Kim, 1988; Khoo, Abu-Rasain, and Homby, 1994; Bradley et al., 1995; Kaczmarek et al., 1994; Sandhu, 1995; Petress, 1995). However, very little has been written about the stress and difficulties experienced by spouses or partners who tend to be more marginalized than the international students and scholars themselves (Verthelyi, 1996, 1994; Schwartz and Kahne, 1993; Vogel, 1986). Moreover, although relationships between social support and physical and mental health have been widely investigated (e.g., Wallston et al., 1983; Gottlieb, 1985; Heitzmann and Kaplan, 1988; Barrera, 1986; Cohen and Wills, 1985; Taylor, 1990), literature has been limited with regard to families of international students who experience stress caused by cultural differences and adaptation, and how service providers may help these individuals cope with their situation. Serious consequences of this isolation include the risk of depression, child abuse, domestic violence, or even suicide (e.g., Vogel, 1986). The international students and families often lack familiarity with service providers and the medical system in the United States, which results in their delayed search for help and the further development of problems.

Structural Difficulties and Gender Roles

Not all of the problems experienced by spouses of international students arise from cultural isolation. Our findings from the focus groups suggest that women who accompany their spouses to the United States are initially prone to be more dependent on their husbands than they were in their home countries. They are seen as wives rather than as individuals. They lack jobs, social status, informal support networks, and extended families, all of which were available at home, and their mental and physical health may therefore become vulnerable. They are in the United States primarily because of their husbands' research or studies, and in their home community they are expected to support their husbands and raise their children rather than to pursue their own interests. The focus groups revealed that the high cost of child care and their nonworking visa status often isolated these women in their apartments with their children. Finally, this particular community is also unique in that there is a very rapid turnover of residents compared to the other ethnic communities and its transience makes it difficult to foster a sense of cohesiveness and community.

PROGRAMMING

Based on these findings, several subprojects have been developed: creating a Web page and information files that contain practical information written in Asian languages; organizing parenting seminars, family orientations, and social gatherings where people with similar needs and interests can meet and create informal networks; planning mental health and well-being seminars; and building collaborative relationships among university subdivisions, i.e., units in the Division of Student Affairs, the School of Social Work, and Department of Psychology. Publicity about the program and its services has also taken place through presentations to groups concerned with women's health, international social work, and other such similar topics.

A major focus of this program has been the development of projects that build on already existing resources in each department, school, or division. For example, both psychology undergraduate students and master of social work (MSW) students have worked on this project as research assistants in exchange for course credits. An undergraduate psychology intern with a focus on community organization and research completed an experiential summer internship for the project. The administrators at the School of Social Work have expressed an interest in developing a community-oriented, internationally focused internship like NCOP, since students who wish to be placed in international social work practicum sites outnumber the available sites.

NCOP has developed a number of methods of reaching out to involve spouses of international students. These methods include visiting Family Housing Language Program English conversation classes to meet spouses and to publicize our programs as well as posting flyers for events in strategic locations, such as the garbage disposal areas, bus stops, and the Community Center at North Campus Family Housing. Second, NCOP organizers have provided services in the languages and cultural contexts of international spouses, rather than just in English and in an "American" way. For example, a seminar about finding baby-sitters also provided names of potential baby-sitters among students in the Department of Asian Languages and Cultures, which helps parents to find baby-sitters who are willing to speak their languages and who understand their cultural contexts better than people found in the classified advertisements of a local newspaper. This seminar also provided on-site translators and transcription of the seminar in three Asian languages.

SURVEY AND PROGRAM DATA

In the summer of 1997, twenty-eight international residents (twenty-six females, two males; average age 31.9) took part in our questionnaire study. All were taking English conversation classes at the Family Housing Language Program during the summer term. Almost all of them were spouses of international students and scholars living in the University of Michigan Family Housing. The intent of this survey was to identify the degree to which our programming addressed the ongoing needs of the community. We were particularly interested in receiving feedback from residents who had not participated in our programs.

The NCOP staff members recruited the respondents on one occasion at the end of a class. Students were given explanations, and only those who agreed to complete the questionnaire stayed in the classroom. The original English questionnaire was translated into Chinese, Japanese, Korean, and Spanish, and the respondents were invited to use the language they were most comfortable with. The questionnaire was five to seven pages long depending on the language, and the time they needed to fill in the questionnaire ranged from approximately ten minutes to twenty minutes. As compensation, those who participated received $5 gift certificates for a nearby supermarket.

RESULTS

Of the participants 15 were Japanese, 12 were Korean, and 1 was German. Ages ranged from 24 to 49 years old; 15 had children, 12 were without, and 1 provided no information with regard to children. Among those who had children, the mean age of the oldest child was 5.6 years old (range .66 to 14 years old), and the mean age for the second child was 6.4 years old (range 0 to 12 years old). Of the respondents 12 identified themselves as their children's primary caregivers, while 3 described somebody else as primary caregiver (spouse/partner/other). The respondents had been in Michigan for an average of 10.4 months with the mode of 12 months (range 1 month to 4 years; 1 case missing). They planned to stay an average of 23 more months in Michigan (mode 12 months, range 5 months to 5 years; 3 cases missing). None identified themselves as being employed; however, 2 respondents were involved in volunteer work. Students at postsecondary level numbered 2 (community college), but the rest did not attend classes outside of the Language Program.

The Hassles Scale (Kanner et al., 1981) was adapted in order to get a sense of the nature and scope of the life stresses experienced by this group. Several items were developed for this population based on findings from the focus groups and previous research on cross-cultural adaptation. The most common hassles identified by the respondents were "trouble reading and writing" (18 people/64 percent), "not undersstanding the language on TV" (17 people/60 percent), "planning/preparing meals" (16 people/57 percent), "friends/relatives far away" (13 people/46 percent), "inability to express oneself " (13 people/46 percent), and "adjusting to the food" (11 people/39 percent). What we can see is that these respondents experience communication as a major stress in their daily lives in the United States (trouble reading and writing, not understanding language on TV, inability to express oneself). Also, dealing with household work around food was perceived as a major hassle (planning/preparing meals, adjusting to the food), perhaps because many women in our study take on the role of preparing meals and assuring their children have a proper diet. In relation to lack of communication ability, not having close friends and relatives around was identified as another major hassle. Together with the open-ended part of the questionnaire, what develops from this picture is that wives, the majority of them mothers, are having trouble understanding English, are experiencing difficulties with making new friends, and thus are unable to gather information through informal networks and through media such as television. Difficulties in buying familiar food, getting used to food distribution systems in the United States, and adjusting to new food also become hassles for these respondents, who are mostly women, since they are often the ones who are responsible for preparing "good" food for their husbands and children.

These results support data from the focus groups we had gathered earlier. They confirm that without language skills, an informal network, and information, these wives experience many layers of difficulties in daily life that may be different from those experienced by their husbands. Although the program has been successful in reaching spouses, these data suggest that many more families could benefit from the program. Outreach to the English language classes may be critical for reaching spouses when they first arrive in family housing.

SYNERGY THROUGH GROUPS

Four types of groups—focus groups, task groups, educational, and mutual aid/self-help groups—are critical elements of the NCOP. Our focus has been on groups because they can be an ideal modality for individual and community empowerment (Gutiérrez and Ortega, 1991; Lee, 1994). Groups can be forums for participation, communication, and community building among program participants. They also provide a means for bringing together the different voices needed for truly multicultural efforts (Gutiérrez et al., 1996).

Our use of focus groups in the initial organizing efforts accomplished both research and program purposes. The focus group modality was used because it allowed us to gather information from multiple perspectives in a relatively brief period of time. This method of research was particularly appealing to our sponsoring organizations because they could meet the multiple goals of gathering data while providing information to residents. These groups also contributed to the visibility of the project. When the community center on North Campus was filled with the voices of Asian women speaking in multiple languages, they demonstrated aurally and visually the constituents we were endeavoring to reach.

The NCOP has been governed by a task group that includes students, faculty, and staff at the university. This task group meets on a monthly basis to assess program progress and plan for the future. In this setting, all participants meet as equals who are committed to the program and the community, although the meetings are facilitated by the students who staff the program. This type of task group format has contributed to the success of the program by building a collaborative process in which different types of expertise and knowledge can be shared. As this is a diverse group in respect to gender, status, and ethnicity, it is also a forum in which our program ideas can be viewed through different lenses. The task group format has been a means to ensure that our research and programming are culturally appropriate.

Educational groups have been the primary method for programming. Programs concerned with parenting, health, and community resources have taken place in the groups. This has permitted us to reach more residents simultaneously and create an environment for community building through participation in group activities. The multilingual nature of this project has required the capacity for simultaneous translation, a critical aspect of these educational groups. In most cases, the primary facilitator or presenter will speak in one language, with student and community volunteers available to translate. This has also allowed the participants to meet various individuals of different nationality groups.

As we move into the second year of this program our plan is to develop more mutual aid/self-help groups. Through our needs and asset assessments we have identified a number of topics and themes that would be amenable for group activities. This includes weekly informal "chat groups" for women who first move to North Campus, discussion groups around parenting and school issues, and groups for families as they prepare to move back to their home countries. Our surveys have identified spouses who are interested in volunteering to plan and implement these programs with other residents. Through this format, we hope to involve residents more directly in the different program components.

SUMMARY

The experiences of international students and their families may seem far from the usual concerns of social workers. However, the experiences of these families are representative of many current and emerging practice realities, such as the influence of global economies, cultural diversity, and the need to prevent physical and mental distress through prevention programs. This program provides a means to develop and evaluate effective methods for multicultural and multilingual community development. As the United States and other countries grow in cultural diversity, these methods will become increasingly important.

Although this chapter has focused on providing services, the focus of this program also involves efforts to affect the structure of the university as well. Administrative support for this project has been tenuous at best and rests on soft moneys and voluntary support. We have encountered questions on our campus about the degree to which "international" and "nonstudent" as well as "family" fall within the legitimate parameters of university service. We have had to share resources such as an office, phone lines, and staff members. Much of the work depends on volunteer work from students, staff, and faculty. Yet, we are often asked from the residents to provide more programs and extend services to nonparent spouses and other international families. For example, Latin American spouses in the Family Housing Language Program have said to us, "It's not fair that you only have things for Asians!" Therefore, we are constantly educating our colleagues about how the struggles of these families are located in the systemic, contextual, familial, and institutional set of forces that affects us all. These efforts have resulted in a two-year grant that will allow us to hire an additional organizer to establish an office in the community and to expand our efforts to other international spouses.

Literature on group work has focused on the relevance of a wide array of social work activity: support, counseling, advocacy, social action, and research. However, theory and practice have often viewed these activities as separate from one another. By creating groups that focus on one activity, such as counseling, to the exclusion of others, we fail to utilize the most exciting potential of group work to act as a catalyst when moving from one level of intervention to the other. We hope that in this chapter we have shared the strategies that have been used to integrate these activities. The NCOP is one way in which principles of cultural competence, empowerment methods, and collaboration among professionals and community participants have converged to meet both individual and social goals through group work.

REFERENCES

Barrera, M., Jr. (1986). Distinctions between social support concepts, measures, and models. *American Journal of Community Psychology,* 14, 413-445.

Bradley, L., Parr, G., Lan, W.Y., Bingi, R., and Gould, L.J. (1995). Counseling expectations of international students. *International Journal for the Advancement of Counseling,* 18, 21-31.

Brown, P. (1994). Participatory research: A new paradigm for social work. In L. Gutiérrez and P. Nurius (Eds.), *Education and Research for Empowerment Practice* (pp. 293-303). Seattle, WA: Center for Policy and Practice Research, University of Washington School of Social Work.

Cohen, S. and Wills, T.A. (1985). Stress, social support, and the buffering hypothesis. *Psychological Bulletin,* 98, 310-357.

Delgado, M. and Humm-Delgado, D. (1982). Natural support systems: Source of strength in Hispanic communities. *Social Work,* 27(1), 83-89.

Gottlieb, B.H. (1985). Social networks and social support: An overview of research, practice, and policy implications. *Health Education Quarterly,* 2, 5-22.

Gutiérrez, L. and Ortega, R. (1991). Developing methods to empower Latinos: The importance of groups. *Social Work with Groups,* 14(2), 23-43.

Gutiérrez, L., Rosegrant Alvarez, A., Nemon, H., and Lewis, E. (1996). Multicultural community organizing: A strategy for change. *Social Work,* 41(5), 501-508.

Heitzmann, C.A. and Kaplan, R.M. (1988). Assessment of methods for measuring social support. *Health Psychology,* 7, 75-109.

Institute of International Education (1995). *Open Doors, 1994-1995.* New York: Author.

Kaczmarek, P., Matlock, G., Merta, R., Ames, M., and Ross, M. (1994). An assessment of international college students' adjustment. *International Journal for the Advancement of Counseling,* 17, 241-247.

Kanner, A., Coyne, J., Schaeffer, C., and Lazarus, R. (1981). Comparison of two modes of stress: Daily hassles and uplifts vs. major life events. *Journal of Behavioral Medicine,* 4, 1-39.

Khoo, P.L.S., Abu-Rasain, M.H., and Homby, G. (1994). Counseling foreign students: A review of strategies. *Counseling Psychology Quarterly,* 7(2), 117-131.

Kim, Y.Y. (1988). *Communication and Cross-Cultural Education: An Integrative Theory.* Philadelphia: Multilingual Matters Ltd.

Lee, J.A.B. (1994). *The Empowerment Approach to Social Work Practice.* New York: Columbia University Press.

Pederson, P. (1995). *The Five Stages of Culture Shock: Critical Incidents Around the World.* Westport, CT: Greenwood Press.

Petress, K.C. (1995). Coping with a new educational environment: Chinese students' imagined interactions before commencing studies in the U.S. *Journal of Instructional Psychology,* 22(1), 59-63.

Sandhu, D.S. (1995). An examination of the psychological needs of the international students: Implications for counseling and psychotherapy. *International Journal for the Advancement of Counseling,* 17, 229-239.

Schwartz, C.G. and Kahne, M.J. (1993). Support for student and staff wives in social transition in a university setting. *International Journal of Intercultural Relations,* 17, 451-463.

Taylor, S. (1990). Health psychology: The science and the field. *American Psychologist,* 45(1), 40-50.

University of Michigan Family Housing (1997). *Family Housing.* Ann Arbor, MI: Author.

University of Michigan Housing International Students Committee (1991). *Meeting the Needs of Foreign Students in Housing: Reports of the Housing International Students Committee.* Ann Arbor, MI: Author.

University of Michigan International Center (1996). *Foreign Student and Staff Statistics: September 1995.* Ann Arbor, MI: Author.

Verthelyi, R.F. (1994). International students' spouses: Invisible sojourners in the culture shock literature. *International Journal of Intercultural Relations,* 19, 387-411.

Verthelyi, R.F. (1996). Facilitating cross-cultural adjustment: A newsletter by and for international students' spouses. *Journal of College Student Development,* 37(6), 699-701.

Vogel, S.H. (1986). Toward understanding the adjustment problems of foreign families in the college community: The case of Japanese wives at the Harvard University Health Services. *Journal of American College Health,* 34, 274-279.

Wallston, B.S., Alagna, S.W., DeVellis, B.M., and DeVellis, R.F. (1983). Social support and physical health. *Health Psychology,* 2, 367-391.

Chapter 9

Families for Reunification: A Mediating Group Model for Birth Parent Self-Assessment

Michael W. Wagner

PARTNERS IN THE PLAN

The provision of services to families whose children are in out-of-home care has been initiated and driven by state and local child welfare law (New York State Social Service Law, §§ 411-424a, 1986) but also operates within the timelines mandated by the Adoption Assistance and Child Welfare Act of 1980 (Public Law 96-272). The dual focus provided by these countervailing legal mandates, one to separate and protect children from abusive and neglectful families and the other to strengthen and unify families, calls upon agencies to develop services and protocols that attempt to balance both sets of values (explicit bibliographies can be found in Azzi-Lessing and Olsen, 1996; Maluccio, Fein, and Olmstead, 1986).

One means of overcoming the limitations imposed by this divided focus for services is to identify ways in which social service practice can build on family strengths to fasten work toward family preservation or reunification. This strengths approach is best articulated by Saleebey (1992), who characterizes social policy as the attempt to build a partnership between the agency and the client. In his assessment of the current state of the profession, Saleebey (1992) suggests that "the legal and political mandates of many agencies, the elements of social control embodied in both the institution and ethos of the agency (strike) a further blow to the possibility of partnership and collaboration between client and helper" (p. 4). Saleebey further notes that a client empowerment stance based on a conscious focus on the clients' strengths is necessary. He notes that while many theoretical perspectives and program developments espouse this philosophical stance, few are able to maintain this focus in the process of client assessment and diagnosis.

This chapter will identify a useful strategy for birth parent group work in an agency context devoted to a strengths approach. It describes a group designed to assist and support birth families in developing a self-assessment of strengths and needs for family reunification. The group model has been developed and piloted at the Children's Aid Society of New York City.

In 1994, the Children's Aid Society, with the support of the New York State Department of Social Services (NYSDSS), instituted an adjustment of the agency's philosophy of service concerning foster parents and birth families. This adjustment took the form of a movement from traditional home finding and foster parent training to a program from the Child Welfare Institute in Atlanta titled the Model Approach to Partnerships in Parenting (MAPP). The MAPP program was selected by the Children's Aid Society as the format for resource parent selection and preparation to meet an anticipated movement toward this program by the NYSDSS, which provided the initial training and support services to agencies choosing to participate. The MAPP Group Preparation and Selection (MAPP/GPS) program provides a framework for the strengths and needs assessment of potential resource families available to foster or adopt children in care out of a home (Bayless and Craig-Oldsen, 1990). The development of the program and its philosophy speaks to the need for the agency workers and the resource parents to work with the birth families to maintain family connections, to build on past attachments, and to promote positive growth and development in children, both emotionally and behaviorally (Bayless and Craig-Oldsen, 1990, Sect. A, p. 5).

The ten-week MAPP/GPS program creates an interactive group experience that allows potential resource families to explore the issues germane to caring for children in out-of-home placement, to assess the family's strengths in the twelve skills needed for resource family effectiveness, to assess the outstanding needs in these twelve skills, and to permit a mutual selection process between agency and family based on strengths. The MAPP/GPS group meets its goals through the use of experiential exercises and family self-assessment in addition to agency assessment of the families. Both resource families and agency workers are encouraged to make efforts to support and serve the needs of birth families in this program; however, a distinct protocol for involving birth family members in the partnership of permanency planning is not identified in the MAPP/GPS protocols. The failure of the program to address fully the issues of birth families points to a significant gap in service that led to the development of the Families for Reunification group.

The strengths-based approach advocated by the MAPP/GPS program rises concurrently with a growing movement in social services as described and reviewed by authors such as Cowger (1994), Hepworth and Larsen (1982), Kisthardt (1992), and Saleebey (1992). Moving from a family dysfunction model of persons in need of services to a client empowerment model, as is championed in these works, allows an agency to take a more direct and active approach to family services by having agency workers and parents work together to develop an assessment of strengths and needs from the client's life perspective (Hepworth and Larsen, 1982). The strengths model is based on the continuing research of the University of Kansas School of Social Welfare (Kisthardt, 1992). The development of a theoretical underpinning for the use of a client-centered assessment model is drawn from the life model of social work practice developed by Germain and Gitterman (1980) and the interactional interdependent model found in the theoretical works of Schwartz (e.g., Schwartz and Zalba, 1971; Schwartz, 1976).

PROGRAM DEVELOPMENT

The establishment of a mutuality process with potential resource parents instigated the idea that birth parents could also be engaged in a similar mutual process. A review of the literature regarding current practice in birth parent groups indicated that mediating model groups (like those developed by Schwartz) were not identified as being used by practitioners. Parent training groups cited in the literature based their work with clients on psychoeducational and Adlerian therapy group models (a review of the relevant literature can be found in Plasse, 1995; Levin, 1992). These group models remain couched in the familiar family dysfunction model with attention to diagnosis, goal-directed behavior, and adjustment in client behavior and attitude. They rise out of organizational group work models (Glasser and Garvin, 1976), functionalist models (Ryder, 1976), or psychosocial group models (Northen, 1976). Other parent training programs are developed in the behavioral therapy models for skill building with parents of "hard to handle" children (a review of relevant literature is found in Magen and Rose, 1994). One might draw such a group out of a task-centered approach to social group work as described by Garvin, Reid, and Epstein (1976). Both of these kinds of interventions, psychoeducational or behavioral groups with birth parents, are based on a deficit model of client assessment and therefore represent the status quo of casework or group work interventions with families. Although both methods have shown certain levels of success in assisting parents in moderating attitudes and changing poor parenting behaviors, they do not invite parents to become a part of their own treatment and planning.

The change of focus as a result of the MAPP/GPS program's impact on the foster care and adoption work of the Children's Aid Society required a new approach be implemented in order to create an atmosphere where agency workers and birth families could also work in a partnership that reflects the overall philosophy that teamwork creates successful conclusions for children in out-of-home placements. The importance of working in partnership as described in MAPP/GPS is an objective that the Children's Aid Society has committed itself to reaching. The effort to have potential resource parents, experienced resource parents, as well as social work staff, support staff, professional staff, and administrative staff attend MAPP groups was one step in building the expectations of the team membership into a pattern that facilitated the goals of the MAPP/GPS model, namely:

> to aid the developmental progress of children, to repair the effects of earlier life experiences or to help children manage the effects of those experiences, to stabilize the relationships of children, to develop strong alliances between the birth families and resource families serving children in care and to strengthen family life. (Bayless and Craig-Oldsen, 1990, Sect. A, pp. 6-7)

The MAPP/GPS model uses the Group Preparation and Selection process to assist families and agencies in making the choice of which potential families will "select in" to become resources to foster children in care or to become resources for adoption. Some families might also "select out" and choose to serve families in some other way. The importance of the group model for mutual support and assistance in the difficult process of "selecting" tells us that if we are also going to work well in partnership with birth families, we will necessarily need to look at a birth family selection process.

As it is currently being used, the model aspires to meet its goals by creating an environment where birth families can make certain gains, but their ongoing needs are left to the traditional foster care casework model where agency workers facilitate and maintain the relationship with the family as a means to encourage partnership. In this context, the actual work of partnership depends deeply on the worker's ability to achieve a working relationship with the birth family at intake. Failure to do so at these initial contacts inhibits rapid and successful reunification and could result in longer placements and more significant injury to family relationships, all of which is clearly against the philosophy of the agency and the MAPP/GPS program.

What a birth family selection process might be, for families involved with the foster care system, could be construed as "selecting in" to join the team working for family reunification by meeting the needs identified by the family and the agency as necessary to diminish the risk of harm or maltreatment of the children, or "selecting out" to assist the team working for family connectedness to assist the children in achieving a statement of permission to remain in out-of-home care and be cared for by a family committed to the children's lives.

What is clear, even at this stage, is that the idea of the birth family selecting in or out is one that is truly foreign to the current state of the system. The concept of birth family selection is one born out of the idea that a committed parent will accomplish those service goals which lead ultimately to discharge from care for the children and their return to the parental home. The family that selects out will choose not to commit to the service goals for a variety of reasons and will allow the child to be adopted. These two options are not simple, nor are they given adequate time in the provision of services to families when the focus of the agency is on the lives of the children as the primary locus for intervention. MAPP/GPS describes this traditional arrangement as when the agency aligns with the children and the parents feel disenfranchised with regard to the decision-making process about the lives of their children. This results in situations of resistance that are commonly described by workers and resource parents alike: birth families do not meet established goals such as visiting children when they say they will or, when visiting, they advise the children to behave in a manner that inhibits the children from fulfilling their own needs. Traditional parenting skills groups, like traditional casework practice, fail to identify the above behavior as representing a family that has not yet chosen to join a partnership to work toward reunification or connection.

PROGRAM DESIGN

In this spirit, a ten-week group for parents working toward reunification was formulated and piloted at the Children's Aid Society in the spring of 1996. Families for Reunification: Partners in the Plan was developed out of a mediating model for group work as described and developed by Schwartz (1976). The group represents a collective of birth parents meeting to provide one another with mutual support as they generate a self-assessment and develop plans for action with the agency regarding permanency planning to reunify with their children. Work in the group is intended to change interaction among the family members and to mediate parents' needs to reunite their families with the need of the agency for planning in order to make reunification a reality. Planning the program based on a mediating model allows for a more successful use of the strengths perspective because the dysfunctional modality of the therapy group in need of curative action (Yalom, 1975) or a parent training group in need of information and a behavioral change, as above, is avoided.

The Families for Reunification group was developed on a ten-week cycle that allows the group to discuss ten strengths demonstrated by families who have been successful in reunifying. These ten strengths are drawn from the MAPP/GPS model specifically to create a common language between agency and families, from the literature, and from common social work practice. The following ten skills were identified for group consideration:

1. *Know your rights:* (Session One) Discussion of the rights and responsibilities of birth parents in working with the agency provides a vehicle to explore the circumstances of placement and steps taken to date to plan for children.

2. *Know your family:* (Session Two) Exploring family histories, stories of childhood, and connections with family members allows for the discovery of family patterns that may be repeating and patterns of isolation that participants might feel.
3. *Be an attachment expert:* (Session Three) Finding an important connection to hold onto with their children, bonding and attachment are discussed to allow participants to see their connections with their children living in the children's attachment with others.
4. *Be a loss expert:* (Session Four) Exploring the behaviors and stages around losses allows participants to identify ways in which their work with the agency may be affected by grief. Reviewing loss histories and considering children's losses moves the group from a past orientation to a more present tense orientation.
5. *Be a family reunion specialist:* (Session Five) In moving into the present, this session represents an opportunity to begin planning improved relationships between parent and child; parent and resource parent; and parent and worker. Focusing on the team aspects of successful visiting planning allows this change.
6. *Manage children's behavior:* (Session Six) Addressing the topic of managing behavior allows participants to discuss some of the issues that trouble them about their children's current behavior as well as about issues concerning the child's being removed from the parent's care. Using a language common to resource parents and workers eases those interactions to promote greater partnership.
7. *Can meet my own needs:* (Session Seven) Many times parents become so intent on the planning for their children's return home that they do not plan to be able to maintain the care they will again give their children. By addressing this topic and challenging participants to identify needs and plans for meeting them, the idea of planning for beyond foster care is made an active part of the group process. Discussion of termination begins in this session.
8. *Maintain a safe and healthy home:* (Session Eight) Parents share many helpful and useful tips for home safety and health planning for their families. The planning focus for reunifica-

tion is strong from this point on in the sessions. Discussions about decisions to make are frequently interspersed with other discussions.

9. *Identify resources in the community:* (Session Nine) Identifying resources for themselves allows a participant to feel a sense of control and self-empowerment in the planning process.

10. *Are partners in permanency planning:* (Session Ten) Termination work with the group comes to fruition in this session and assessments of the ten skill areas are repeated and written down in session. Participants leave the group with a written assessment in their own words meant to better assist them in joining with their worker in a strengths-based permanency plan.

Each skill area was addressed by the group during the weekly meetings and discussions, exercises, and journal work of the group members. Discussions were open for participants to share their thoughts and concerns in each of the topic areas as well as the ongoing process of working with the agency to reunify with their children. Exercises and journal suggestions were presented in keeping with topics to allow for work during the week to identify strengths and needs. In addition, group members were asked each week to identify a strength that they had in the skill area discussed in that week's session. Strength statements were identified in sentences such as "I have a strength! In Session Five we talked about the skill Be a Family Reunion Specialist, and I identified a strength. I show that I am a family reunion specialist because I . . ."

Participants would then identify one or more ways in which they demonstrate strength in that area. This use of a self-identification model allowed the participant to become directly involved in the work of mutually coming to understand and see the strengths they bring to their situation as well as allowing for a concrete representation of the group discussions. One parent asked assistance in recording this material and said, "I am because I meet with (my child) every week now instead of every other week." Group members assisted one another in identifying strengths and encouraged others to identify their own strengths.

Parents were also asked weekly to identify needs in relation to the different skill areas. A need statement was developed in the same way as the strength statement, and parents were asked to think about the things they would like to be able to do or learn in their preparation for working in partnership. An example of a need statement:

> I have a need. In Session Five we talked about the skill Be a Family Reunion Specialist, and I identified a need. In order to be a family reunion specialist, I need to *talk with my worker about having my visits earlier so that my baby isn't napping during the visit time.*

Parents assisted one another in identifying needs and participated in some of the problem solving necessary to meet the group's needs. The development of the mutual aid process and the functioning of the group as a mediating force between the parents and the agency made this task particularly important (see appendix for an overview of the ten strength/need statements for Families for Reunification).

The arrangement of weekly group topics was designed to coincide with the anticipated growth of the group's cohesiveness and increased interpersonal connectedness. Sessions One, Two, and Three are memory intensive, asking parents to recall and recount their stories, to tell about the placement of their children and the unfairness of a system that removes children from families. It is an opportunity for parents to talk about their families, their histories, their children, and to begin to explore the experience of their children's placement. Journal work includes a family-gram, stories of their childhood, and plans for maintaining attachments. Materials and activities in these sessions are drawn from the group and from Gildner (1994, Module 1, pp. 27-34, and Module 2, pp. 80-92) and Plasse (1995).

Session Four stands alone as an opportunity to delve into the deeper issues of personal loss. Parents are presented with the idea that grief and grief behavior stands in the way of their ability to plan for their children. Discussions of the stages of grieving and the idea of cycling back through grief are encouraged. Adaptations from the seminal work of Elisabeth Kübler-Ross (1975) provide the theoretical basis for this session. Parents are asked to review their loss histories and to begin to look at whether there are strengths in loss to be discovered now that they are able to reflect on them. Parents are also reminded that their children are also suffering a loss and will still be grieving that loss upon return home. These concepts and practices are drawn from Kübler-Ross (1978) and from Gildner (1994, Module 2, pp. 51-63).

Sessions Five, Six, and Seven are developed to provide immediate information for parents as they continue to work with the agency while their children are still in care. Parents are encouraged to visit their children and to make visits useful and productive for the sake of permanency planning as well as for themselves. Materials regarding family visitation strategies were adapted from Hess and Proch (1988). Managing behaviors is presented to begin impacting on the strategies that parents have already used to discipline their children and to be able to give them opportunities to explore and attempt new ways of doing things. In an effort to create symmetry for this session the "Fifteen Skills for Managing Behavior" list from the MAPP/GPS program is used (Gildner, 1994, Module 2, pp. 112-118). Parents are challenged to meet their own needs especially while their children are in care, to look deep and discover what they want for themselves so that decisions to reunify are based on strengths (specific intervention strategies are adapted from Arnold, 1978). All of these skills are germane to the permanency planning process as they form the basis for casework assessments of the clients in their interactions with the children.

In Sessions Eight and Nine the group begins looking toward the conclusion of their children's placements and begins to identify those strengths and needs that are present for the children returning home. Self-assessing their homes for safety and health and identifying those resources which they and their children will need when discharge occurs allows parents to prepare for their own self-judgment as a part of their planning process.

Session Ten is set aside as a graduation to a new way of interacting with the agency and the family's caseworker. Parents recomplete all nine previous assessments on the skills and, in addition, identify strengths for being partners in the planning process for their children and obstacles that may keep them from a full partnership. Parents are encouraged to share their self-assessments with their workers as a part of this partnership as well as to use their assessments to document their own progress in work at family court and with the public child welfare agencies.

ANALYSIS

This original group had been designed for and offered to 12 partici-pants and was attended by 8 parents (7 females and 1 male). Of the par-ticipants, 7 consented to complete questionnaires at the end of the series. Of these 7, 4 had attended groups previously. They repre-sented a range of ages from 24 to 44 with a mean of 32.9 years of age. Their children had been in care a range of 0.5 years to 4 years with a mean of 2.14 years and a median of 1.5 years. The 8 participants at-tended an average of 8 of the 10 meetings despite frequent court and medical appointments, and all but 1 member completed their self-as-sessments in Session Ten. These participants completed the group in June 1996. They all continue to work with the agency and several are in the final stages of discharge of their children from care, although none are yet completed.

Group members completed a consumer satisfaction questionnaire anonymously, which represents the only data on group functioning gathered to date. Of the 7 respondents, 86 percent felt that the 10 skills identified were the most important topics (4 of 7 strongly agreed). All 7 felt that the material discussed in group could be used immediately with their children even though their children remained in foster care. All 7 members felt that the in-group discussions were helpful in making plans for their children. Of the 7, 28 percent felt that their plans for their children had not changed as a result of the group experience, while 42 percent felt that they had made changes in their plans. As a consumer satisfaction tool, more so than an outcome assessment, this questionnaire has not been subjected to rigorous va-lidity testing, but the results gained indicated that all of the parents who responded felt the group should be provided to other families and that its focus is specific and useful.

An assessment of the impact of the group on permanency planning behaviors is under development and will be implemented with future groups. These instruments are hoped to produce some data to support the emerging sense that the process of doing a self-assessment and the use of a parent's group modality within the permanency planning process are both useful and beneficial to group members and to the agency. Pre- and postgroup questionnaires along with a tracking tool to identify those attendees who are successful in reunifying in comparison with the general population would provide at least a hint of the usefulness of the group.

Questionnaires to assess worker relationships with their birth families in casework contacts are being devised to determine if the goal of generating a working partnership for planning has been met. Families who had attended the group could then be compared in subjective interview situations with their caseworkers with birth parents who had not attended the group to determine whether group participants engage in more "partnership" activities than do those parents who do not attend. Pre- and postmeasures of these sorts of partnership behaviors would provide comparisons and contrasts for further study.

Assessment of this group process from an outcome standpoint would be premature. The mediating model from which the program was developed does not allow for the discrete assessment of "the group's" intervention apart from the work of the individual parent or the work of the agency. The focus and goal of the group is to promote a more active and equal partnership between parents, resource parents, and agency workers.

One assessment that is already available, however, is to determine whether this group design meets the desired development of a strengths-based intervention for birth families whose children are in out-of-home care. Saleebey (1992, pp. 5-8) identifies assumptions and prerequisites for strengths-based interventions as respect of client's strengths, multiplicity of client's strengths, client motivation based on fostering strengths, social worker as a collaborator with the client (avoid a "victim" mind-set), and identification of an environment full of resources.

According to Schwartz (1976), the power of the group lies in its ability to assist the members as they operate in the many environments and systems in which they find themselves. This is especially important when a family suffers the crisis of the removal of the children. It is also a time when a parent's ability to advocate for self is impaired by the shock, grief, and anger inherent in the removal of the children. The Families for Reunification group deals with this fragile time with all of the supports of a strengths perspective.

Based on the idea that a client's self-assessment is a more valuable tool for both the client and the agency than one more worker's assessment, the group immediately generates a climate in which the client's rights are respected and it is relatively easy to identify strengths in the ten areas crucial to successful outcomes for the parents. This focus on client strengths allows the group to provide a motivating environment for the partnership that the agency ethos is reaching out to provide with the parent. In this and all mediating groups, the worker appears as a collaborator in the process. "His (or her) moves are directed towards specific purposes, limited in scope and time, and touching only those within his (or her) immediate environment," while the group is "a project in mutual aid, focused on certain specific problems, and set within a larger system—the agency—whose function is to provide help with just such problems" (Schwartz, 1976, p. 185). The group at the center of this process avoids a victimization through connection with others. This connectedness helps all members to discover the resources in environments thought to be empty, the strengths where none were perceived, and the hope where only despair remained. Figure 9.1 depicts the mediating model for group work.

Saleebey (1992, pp. 8-13) also identifies the key concepts that create the strengths perspective. These concepts also must be assessed against the model: empowerment, membership, regeneration and healing from within, synergy, dialogue, and collaboration and suspension of disbelief.

Partnership is an embodiment of empowerment because it calls on both parties to have expectations of each other and to make them explicit. The Families for Reunification group design relates to the "easy" client who has no difficulty meeting permanency planning goals and the focus on work outside the group allows even the infre-

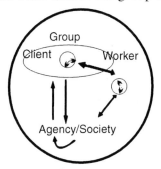

FIGURE 9.1. The Mediating Model for Group Work Practice (*Source:* Adapted from Schwartz, 1976, p. 184.)

quent attendee to benefit from the assessment work that is done. Discussions in the group about the attitudes society has about parents whose children are in care speak to the parents' feelings of isolation and powerlessness. One member stated, "I'm not one of those mothers who is starving her kids. But that's how I'm treated." The early sessions seek to explore the "power within themselves, their families and their neighborhoods" (Saleebey, 1992, p. 9).

The use of the mediating group and the process of self-assessment produce a sense of membership that is unavailable to the parent in individual casework counseling. In the group, the members tell their stories and receive encouragement from others, are encouraged by one another in their successes and efforts, and find links with one another and their communities through the mutual aid process.

A social agency can do little to avoid the tendency of the professional social service sector to diagnose and in a way rob clients of the dignity of their own strengths. Group members speak of the diagnoses that have been placed on them in their process through the child welfare system and many comments echo the words of a group member who said, "I talked about myself and they used it against me." Rather than continue on in this vein, the assessments from this group model arise from the clients themselves and the worker makes it clear that the worker's function is to facilitate the process and not to elaborate a concurrent assessment. Developing the final assessment in Session Ten represents a movement toward healing from within.

Development of materials that allow for the greatest possible group interaction recognizes the importance of synergy. "[W]hen phenomena . . . are brought into interrelationship, they create new and often unexpected patterns and resources that typically exceed the complexity of their individual constituents" (Saleebey, 1992, p. 11). Each group served will develop its own patterns and its own specific artifacts built out of its own synergy. This synergy is the first step of movement back into the life of a community and an end to some families' isolation. One parent who described herself as being basically alone, without family or community support, discovered within the group support structure a continuing supportive friendship with another group member. This parent relates that the two continue to speak by phone and that she feels less isolated.

Groups are by their very definition opportunities for dialogue and collaboration. Members develop within the group environment the ability to share closely held beliefs, to struggle with the pain of past and present losses, to respond to other people's ideas, and to receive responses to their ideas. Saleebey (1992) suggests that "[we] can only come into being through a creative and emergent relationship with the external world" (p. 11).

Most critically, the Families for Reunification group creates an opportunity for a suspension of disbelief, truly a rare opportunity in social work practice. In a system full of people demanding concrete proof for every statement these parents make, the group provides a personal opportunity for these parents to frame their experiences in their own way. Parents engaged in this process are sometimes so surprised by the fact that the worker is not "checking up" on the responses by reviewing case records or gathering separate information about members that they challenge the worker's commitment to the group. In a recent session, a member asked if the worker was going to write an assessment of the individual members. When the worker replied that the group members were to write their own assessments, the member responded, "Well, what good will that do us?" The discussion that followed focused on the truth that workers always write the assessments that are used to make decisions about individual cases. The worker went on to state, "You all are going to be able to go into your caseworker's office with your own paperwork, your own assessments, and your own goals. How many parents do that?" The member sat back and, as the rest of the members began to murmur, relaxed and commented, "Where was this group eight months ago when my children were taken away?" All parents struggle with the idea that their assessments will not be of any use. By maintaining a focus on the purpose of the group, creating a partnership, the worker assists the members in identifying strengths that help them to meet with their caseworkers and the agency in a planning perspective.

CONCLUSION

Families for Reunification: Partners in the Plan continues to be a newly formed group. Its effectiveness for speeding reunification services and for improving client-worker interactions to meet planning goals is yet to be fully assessed. Consumer satisfaction surveys suggest that parents found the group beneficial and that their strengths had been recognized by the agency. Continuing follow-up with these families, development of an ongoing support group to continue the progress from the original groups, and more series of the group are necessary before more certain data can be presented to support this emerging sense of a successful group design.

The MAPP/GPS model and the philosophical change that it represents provide an opportunity for the Children's Aid Society to embrace this strengths perspective more fully, benefiting the lives of children and families even when those families are separated by the neglectful or abusive behavior of birth parents. The Families for Reunification group represents the fullest expression of this strengths perspective by taking on the mediating function of group intervention to assist parents and agency workers in developing a working partnership. Agencies hoping to make the key concepts of a strengths perspective more than simple buzzwords must endeavor to develop supportive programs such as the Families for Reunification group. This will provide opportunities for clients to join in a mutual aid process for the discovery and practice of individual client strengths, to clarify their own sense of the problems leading to the need for services, to find healing from within, to use strengths to meet their needs, and to develop the courage to hope for a future where they are active participants in the plans for their own lives. This is the essence of client empowerment and it must emerge in the interaction between the clients, the workers, and the agency in order to impact the families and the society in which they live.

APPENDIX:
FAMILIES FOR REUNIFICATION—
PARTNERS IN THE PLAN, FINAL ASSESSMENT

Everyone has strengths which make us who we are. By identifying our strengths we prepare ourselves to be partners in the permanency plan of our children.

In Session One we talked about the skill *know your rights,* and I identified a strength: "I show that I know my rights by . . ."

In Session Two we talked about the skill *know your family,* and I identified a strength: "I show that I know my family because I know . . ."

In Session Three we talked about the skill *be an attachment expert,* and I identified a strength: "I show that I am an attachment expert because I . . ."

In Session Four we talked about the skill *be a loss expert,* and I identified a strength: "I show that I am a loss expert because I . . ."

In Session Five we talked about the skill *be a family reunion specialist,* and I identified a strength: "I show that I am a family reunion specialist because I . . ."

In Session Six we talked about the skill *manage children's behavior,* and I identified a strength: "I show that I can manage children's behavior because I . . ."

In Session Seven we talked about the skill *meet my own needs,* and I identified a strength: "I show that I can meet my own needs because I . . ."

In Session Eight we talked about the skill *make a safe and healthy home,* and I identified a strength: "I show that I can maintain a healthy home because I . . ."

In Session Nine we talked about the skill *identify resources in the community,* and I identified a strength: "The resource that I have identified in my community is: . . ."

All people have needs. We identify our needs so that we can join in the process of permanency planning for our children by setting our goals for personal growth.

In Session One we talked about the skill *know your rights,* and I identified a need: "I need to . . ."

In Session Two we talked about the skill *know your family,* and I identified a need: "I need to . . ."

In Session Three we talked about the skill *be an attachment expert,* and I identified a need: "To be an attachment expert I need to . . ."

In Session Four we talked about the skill *be a loss expert,* and I identified a need: "To be a loss expert I need to . . ."

In Session Five we talked about the skill *be a family reunion specialist,* and I identified a need: "To be a family reunion specialist I need to . . ."

In Session Six we talked about the skill *manage children's behavior,* and I identified a need: "To manage children's behavior I need to . . ."

In Session Seven we talked about the skill *meet my own needs,* and I identified a need: "To meet my own needs I need to . . ."

In Session Eight we talked about the skill *make a safe and healthy home,* and I identified a need: "To maintain a healthy home I need to . . ."

In Session Nine we talked about the skill *identify resources in the community,* and I identified a need: "I must still find a resource to provide me with . . ."

In Session Ten, we are talking about the skill *be a partner in permanency planning.* To be a partner in my plan, I commit to using these strengths that I have identified to meet my needs. My signature to this assessment is my commitment.

In Session Ten, we talk about the skill *be a partner in permanency planning.* I have identified a need that keeps me from working in partnership: "To meet this need I will . . ."

REFERENCES

Arnold, L.E. (Ed.) (1978). *Helping Parents Help Their Children.* New York: Brunner/Mazel.

Azzi-Lessing, L. and Olsen, L.J. (1996). Substance abuse affected families in the child welfare system: New challenges, new alliances. *Social Work,* 41(1), 15-23.

Bayless, L. and Craig-Oldsen, H.L. (1990). *Model Approach to Partnerships in Parenting: Group Preparation and Selection of Foster and/or Adoptive Parents Implementation Guidebooks* (Fourth Edition). Atlanta, GA: Child Welfare Institute.

Cowger, C.D. (1994). Assessing client strengths: Clinical assessment for client empowerment. *Social Work,* 39(3), 262-268.

Garvin, C.D., Reid, W., and Epstein, L. (1976). A task-centered approach. In R.W. Roberts and H. Northen (Eds.), *Theories of Social Work with Groups* (pp. 238-267). New York: Columbia University Press.

Germain, C. and Gitterman, A. (1980). *The Life Model of Social Work Practice.* New York: Columbia University Press.

Gildner, M. (1994). *An Overview of the Group Preparation and Selection of Resource Families: Leader's Guide* (Modules 1-3). Atlanta, GA: Child Welfare Institute.

Glasser, P.H. and Garvin, C.D. (1976). An organizational model. In R.W. Roberts and H. Northen (Eds.), *Theories of Social Work with Groups* (pp. 75-115). New York: Columbia University Press.

Hepworth, D.H. and Larsen, J.A. (1982). *Direct Social Work Practice*. Belmont, CA: Wadsworth.

Hess, P.M. and Proch, K.O. (1988). *Family Visiting in Out-of-Home Care: A Guide to Practice*. Washington, DC: Child Welfare League of America.

Kisthardt, W.E. (1992). A strength model of case management: The principles and functions of a helping partnership with persons with persistent mental illness. In D. Saleebey (Ed.), *The Strengths Perspective in Social Work Practice* (pp. 59-83). White Plains, NY: Longman.

Kübler-Ross, E. (1975). *On Death and Dying*. New York: MacMillan.

Kübler-Ross, E. (1978). Helping parents teach their children about death and life. In L.E. Arnold (Ed.), *Helping Parents Help Their Children* (pp. 270-278). New York: Brunner/Mazel.

Levin, A.E. (1992). Groupwork with parents in the family foster care system: A powerful method of engagement. *Child Welfare, 71*(5), 457-473.

Magen, R.H. and Rose, S.R. (1994). Parents in groups: Problem solving versus behavioral skills training. *Research on Social Work Practice, 4*(2), 172-191.

Maluccio, A.N., Fein, E., and Olmstead, K.A. (1986). *Permanency Planning for Children: Concepts and Methods*. New York: Tavistock.

Northen, H. (1976). Psychosocial practice in small groups. In R. Roberts and H. Northen. *Theories of Social Work with Groups* (pp. 116-152). New York: Columbia University Press.

Plasse, B.R. (1995). Parenting groups for recovering addicts in a day treatment center. *Social Work, 40*(1), 65-74.

Ryder, E.L. (1976). A functional approach. In R.W. Roberts and H. Northen (Eds.), *Theories of Social Work with Groups* (pp. 153-170). New York: Columbia University Press.

Saleebey, D. (1992). Introduction: Power in the people. In D. Saleebey (Ed.), *The Strengths Perspective in Social Work Practice* (pp. 3-26). White Plains, NY: Longman.

Schwartz, W. (1976). Between client and system: The mediating function. In R.W. Roberts and H. Northen (Eds.), *Theories of Social Work with Groups* (pp. 171-197). New York: Columbia University Press.

Schwartz, W. and Zalba, S.R. (Eds.) (1971). *The Practice of Group Work*. New York: Columbia University Press.

Yalom, I. (1975). *The Theory and Practice of Group Psychotherapy*. New York: Basic Books.

Chapter 10

Efficacy of Group Interventions with Seriously Mentally Ill Parents: A Literature Review

Gordon MacDonald

INTRODUCTION

The issues of parenting and child rearing for the seriously mentally ill population have surfaced recently as a result of social policy changes over the past few decades, shifting direction from that of segregation and isolation of the mentally ill to that of integration and inclusion. Garvin (1992) acknowledges that "their disability is severe and involves significant handicaps in fulfilling the requirements of . . . familial roles. . . . The need for new services for this population is great and has been intensified as a result of the process of deinstitutionalization" (p. 67). Individuals diagnosed with a major mental illness, such as schizophrenia, and those who also have parenting roles and responsibilities, require intervention and assistance. Papell (1992) supports these notions, stating, "If these are the new populations we are to address, then as group workers we must search out some very specific knowledge and we must certainly talk about outreach, prevention, education, empowerment as well as treatment" (p. 23). Coping with the normal routines and demands of parenting when one's life is overlaid with the debilitating consequences of a mental illness is a monumental task that is often difficult to achieve. Seeman (1996) writes:

A comprehensive treatment approach to the woman with schizophrenia includes individual and group therapies, family counselling, carefully monitored pharmacotherapy, attention to income supplementation, adequate housing, vocational assistance, educational upgrading, social and life skills training, emphasis on general health and meaning of life issues. (p. 196)

This chapter is a review of the literature regarding the efficacy of group interventions with parents who have a serious mental illness. The chapter is organized as follows: First, a review of the population will provide a context of prevalence, characteristics and features, and the treatment difficulties of parents with a serious mental illness. Second, a comprehensive review of the literature written over the past decade, specific to the nature and efficacy of group interventions with seriously mentally ill parents, will provide a level of awareness regarding the quantity, quality, and effectiveness of group modalities. Finally, the implications emerging from the literature review will be discussed as an effort to heighten consciousness and sensitivity to the issues facing parents with serious mental illness, child protection agencies, service providers, and policymakers. The conclusion will provide a brief summary of the review and include broad-based recommendations for the future.

DEFINITION OF A GROUP

Many descriptions and definitions of a group exist, even within the discipline of social work. Gitterman (1986) builds on the mutual aid concept of Schwartz (1961), describing the investment of individuals within this mutual aid system: "As people develop comfort in being together and a greater openness to examine their perceptions and behaviors, they simultaneously develop a sense of collective strength and power" (p. 32). Lee (1986) builds on Germain and Gitterman's (1980) life model, indicating that

[t]he points of intervention are located throughout the life cycle both before, during and after trouble arises. It may have a social action, socialization or more insight oriented and support focus. It is a broad model reaching people where they live and offering mutual aid. (p. 47)

Schwartz (1986) continues to develop his concept of a group in this description:

Its deeper truth lays in its vision of a relationship in which the qualities of leadership are expressed in the joys of human collaboration, rather than in the action of the knower on the naive, the strong on the weak, the expert on the uninitiated. (p. 23)

Schwartz (1986) continues, "there was something in the nature of doing, and particular collective doing, that helped people find new ways of looking at themselves and the world around them" (p. 24). Kurland and Salmon (1996) build on Schwartz's notions, stating that group work is "a process where mutual aid is central and maximized . . . it is the quality of the mutual aid process that occurs in a group that is central in distinguishing social group work practice from other group efforts" (p. 25).

Middleman and Wood (1995) describe the group as "the ideal medium for consciousness raising. It is an intimate and mutually supportive situation for discussion of lived traumas, for examination of the relationship between individual experience and political ascription, and for subsequent social action" (p. 11). Falck (1995) suggests there are a number of criteria that determine social work with groups. The following are a few of the criteria he considers to be relevant:

- Clients teach one another (i.e., learn from one another) how to meet their human needs through a democratic group process.
- The aim of social group work activity is to assist clients to teach one another.
- Clients learn from one another as well as from and through the worker how to bring about change outside their group.
- Clients are constantly helped to become conscious of the ethically and scientifically documented fact that the behaviors of all persons have significant consequences for others, both inside and outside the group. (p. 69)

Garvin (1997) identifies the group as a medium to improve social functioning, suggesting that the purpose and use of groups is socialization. Social functioning problems can be improved through many content forms such as recreation, education, and issue-specific topics.

The threads of commonality in these definitions are the benchmarks and filters of understanding used in this review of the literature.

Because of the scarcity of material related to the topic, the literature reviewed goes beyond the discipline of social work. In this regard, the definitions of a group as previously outlined do not always aptly apply to those groups referred to in the studies; however, the definitions are useful for contrast and comparison to the variety of group applications uncovered in this review. It is also noted that the language and terminology in this chapter have medical and pathology overtones. This is not intended to minimise the values and principles behind social work with groups; rather, it is a reflection of the existing literature and the venues where many of these groups meet.

THE POPULATION

Prevalence

It is estimated that 50 percent of individuals with a serious mental illness are mothers and fathers living with their children (Nadelson, 1996). It is further estimated that 50 percent of children living with a parent with a serious mental illness will have, to some degree, maladjustment problems (Gangbar, 1997; Pound, 1996). The possibility of someone in the population having schizophrenia is about one in 100. If one parent has schizophrenia, the chance of a child having schizophrenia is 10 to 13 percent, and if both parents have schizophrenia, the risk is increased to four in ten (Cohler, Stott, and Musik, 1996; Gottesman, 1991; Halgin and Whitbourne, 1993; Rubovits, 1996). Only a minority of women, approximately 25 to 45 percent, and a larger proportion of men, 60 percent, with serious mental illness do not marry, leaving up to 75 percent of women and 40 percent of men with marital status (Mowbray et al., 1995; Bachrach and Nadelson, 1988). Seeman (1996) writes that "many young people with schizophrenia, especially young women, are motivated to become parents and will do so even when seriously ill and unsupported" (p. 190). Coverdale and Aruffo (1989) and Zemencuk, Rogosch, and Mowbray (1995) concur that seriously mentally ill women are sexually active and have a greater than average number of children.

Parents with serious mental illness are in compounded risk situations involving themselves and their children (McNamee, Lipman, and Hicks, 1995; Wang and Goldschmidt, 1994). Demographic and descriptive features provide an important understanding of this population and help to highlight the complexities of intervention strategies, specifically group interventions, applied to these unique individuals. Features of this population are discussed in the following section.

Features

It cannot be assumed that the needs of parents or children are being met if a parent has a serious mental illness. Many studies indicate that long-term support is a necessity for these families because neither parents nor children are able to cope with the dynamics and demands specific to the situations where major mental illness is involved (Cook and Cohler, 1986; Dunn, 1993; Penn and Meuser, 1996). Families become increasingly isolated over time and require a number of buffering supports that act as protective factors against continuing deterioration: network supports, symptom control, and an adequate level of caretaking for the children involved (Gangbar, 1997).

As a group, children of psychologically troubled parents report greater personal distress than children of the psychologically well (Cohler, Stott, and Musik, 1996). Children with a schizophrenic parent show multiple cognitive, attentional, and social impairments. They also experience delays in language, maintain immature modes of communication, and distance themselves from parental attachment. Parental psychopathology may be communicated to the child, leading to impairments in attachments and reality testing. A diminished capacity to stimulate the child also may lead to developmental delays (Cook and Cohler, 1986; Goodman and Brumley, 1990; Hamilton, Jones, and Hammon, 1993; Rubovits, 1996; Weintraub, 1987).

Responding to the responsibilities and obligations surrounding the tasks of parenting is stressful and conflictual. These parents are often resentful about giving to their children with whom they spend more time in protest than in play (Field, Healy, and Goldstein, 1988). Primitive emotional needs often limit their ability to negotiate interpersonal relationships, especially with regard to maintaining closeness. Sustaining a marital relationship or developing a new partnership is a perpetual struggle. Seriously mentally ill parents are also restricted in their ability to differentiate their needs from those of the child, making it difficult to accurately assess the child's needs and to determine the dangers and boundaries for the child in their shared environment.

Perceptions of their child's abilities are often distorted and fewer interactions with the child contribute to the difficulties related to parenting (Goodman and Brumley, 1990; Rubovits, 1996).

All of these factors signal failure for the parent with a mental illness. In Western culture particularly, "[p]arenthood is the greatest developmental challenge of adult life, and failure to function adequately as a parent is the most shame-ridden of adult failures, the loss least amenable to integration" (Gopfert, Webster, and Seeman, 1996, p. 3).

Parenting is a high-stakes task for parents with a serious mental illness. The illness inhibits natural abilities to cope with parenting duties and it also magnifies the consequences of inadequate parenting. Parents who are handicapped with a serious mental illness are further judged by a society that casts shame on them for an impairment beyond their control. Many of the aspects of this population present difficulties for the intervention and treatment process, as presented in the following section.

Difficulties Specific to Group Intervention

Three key difficulties regarding group interventions with this population include isolation, lack of interpersonal skills and response to treatment, and the degree of cooperation and commitment. Each of these difficulties requires an array of strategies to overcome the negative impact of these dynamics as a prerequisite to functioning in a group context and as a requisite to maintaining the ability to function within a group context (Kanas, 1991). Consideration of these factors promotes an appreciation for the complexities of this population and helps us in developing an understanding about the enormous hurdles these individuals have to overcome in their struggle to belong.

Isolation may be represented by a lack of trust or paranoia regarding the helping profession, group members, and authorities or may perhaps be the result of a lack of confidence and self-esteem (Kanas, 1991). Isolation may also be seen as a response to minimise the fear of losing their child. Possessiveness and overprotectiveness of a child against apprehension may be motivating factors to limit contact with others. A group intervention may be very anxiety provoking for a paranoid, untrusting individual or for the person struggling to gain confidence. For the overprotective parent, disclosure of parenting problems or asking for help may be inhibited by the fear of losing a child.

Lack of interpersonal skills may restrict the interactive process necessary for group functioning. An individual who is capable of addressing only his or her own emotional needs has a limited ability to listen, develop emotional connections, and empathise with others. An inability to judge, pick up on social cues, and communicate consistently requires a repetition of learning opportunities that may limit the amount of parenting-related items a group of this nature is capable of processing at a given time. Difficulties in maintaining relationships may also be a restrictive factor for group development.

The final aspect of treatment difficulties relates to cooperation, commitment, and response to treatment. Denial, inability to cope with the illness, and displeasure with the responsibilities of being a parent are all important issues to resolve in the course of treatment. A group intervention may serve to create a level of agitation and further resistance to treatment if an individual has not expressed a readiness to participate. The intensity and frequency of a group format may become an anxiety factor rather than a support factor and may contribute to the individuals' frustration if a group is seen as just another expectation in a series of other interventions or agency involvement. The lack of commitment for long-term continuity of the program may also limit the level of participants' commitment.

Breton (1985) describes these individuals as hard to reach: nonseekers, unresponsive, unpredictable, or uninvolved. She qualifies her labelling by indicating that individuals behave resistantly or accommodatingly because they are motivated towards a particular goal. Breton's suggestion for group workers is to start with people's motivation; to demonstrate competence by doing for or with the individual before asking them to do for themselves; to create optimal challenges or reasonable opportunities for success; and to use the individuals' natural support networks. On the other hand, Garvin (1992) indicates that individuals have opportunities in a group context that provides a safe and accepting setting to acquire and practice social behaviors. In this sense, it is the safe milieu of a group that encourages participation. Perhaps both arguments are relevant when assessing responses to treatment.

It is important to consider these factors as unique to this population and their relevance to the use of a group intervention in addressing parenting concerns. Group interventions designed to help restore and maintain parenting functions are discussed in the following review of literature.

SERIOUSLY MENTALLY ILL PARENTS AND GROUP INTERVENTION

There are three main target populations where group interventions are used with the seriously mentally ill. Specific to schizophrenia, the individual client has been identified as needing a group response within the context of an overall treatment plan (Seeman, 1996). The second population identified is comprised of the families of individuals with schizophrenia. Numerous studies indicate the importance of a family system in the effective treatment of schizophrenia (Gidron, Gutterman, and Hartman, 1990; Hogarty et al., 1986; Kane, DiMartino, and Jiminez, 1990; Kassis, Boothroyd, and Ben-Dror, 1990; Leff et al., 1989; Walsh, 1987). The third population identified is parents with a serious mental illness. This is not specific to schizophrenia alone. The two main diagnoses of this parent population are schizophrenia and depression. Given the high incidence of depression associated with schizophrenia (40 percent), the applicability of the literature related to parents with a serious mental illness seems relevant to the schizophrenic population (Gangbar, 1997). Reference to serious mental illness and schizophrenia may be used interchangeably within this chapter.

The majority of group interventions with seriously mentally ill parents include the children as components of the treatment process. The applications of the group modality include parent-child groups, child groups, and parent groups. Varying types of objectives, content, and process are used within each of these groups based on the perceived needs of the participants involved and the mandates of the agencies providing the services. For the purpose of this chapter, the concentration of study is specific to the efficacy of parent groups for the seriously mentally ill because they are impacted with unique problems that go beyond treatment. These problems, for example, child welfare legislation, may impede interventions. It is recognised, however, that the combination of treatment applications provides the greatest effect (Seeman, 1996).

Studies and Applications

Project CHILD in Providence, Rhode Island, targeted parent functioning and rehabilitation; the cognitive, emotional, and social development of the child; and the optimisation of the parent-child relationship as its main sphere of intervention. The project's goals were to improve parenting skills and to remedy developmental delays in children, particularly with regard to language, attention, attachment, and separation. Medication, supportive individual therapy, and home visits were provided as supplements to an intensive, three-day-per-week program for mothers and children. The program included a teaching time with mother and child, a lunch program, a social club for mothers, stimulation groups for toddlers and preschoolers, transportation, and community liaison (Rubovits, 1996).

The notion of the "group as life" described by Lang (1997) appears to be a complementary description of this program. Lang's model promotes the life of a group as a natural unfolding of events relevant to the members. It is not a fabricated package of interventions or exercises geared toward changing individuals; rather, the model's advantage is that it moves, turns, and sways with the feelings, expressions, needs, and wishes of the members as they experience life together and use these life experiences as opportunities for developing insight, growth, and change. Components of the group time in Project CHILD are indicative of natural patterns of daily structure, interaction, and networking skills. There is little anecdotal or empirical evidence of the success of this program or the efficacy of the parent group intervention given by Rubovits (1996) in the description of the program.

NEWPIN in London, England, is a voluntary organisation that targets families with no community support. The thrust of its efforts is the prevention of child abuse through the use of individual counselling and group therapy interventions for parents. The group modality is intended to provide therapeutic support, teach alternate ways of relating, build self-esteem and trust, address issues of loss and separation due to relationship breakdowns, and respond to issues of personal well-being (Jenkins, 1996).

Efficacy of the group intervention was measured on the basis of improved self-esteem, personal relationships, and general mental health. No data were provided to substantiate the degree of effect nor were methodologies and discussions included in the article. It is interesting to note that Jenkins (1996) made a specific point about group culture. There was a deliberate attempt to maintain a nucleus of mothers to carry on the group culture and offer the model to new mothers. Although the authors did not identify any particular theory, culture in the sense that it was mentioned may be interpreted as a level of cohesiveness and nominative structure that identifies these individuals as an autonomous group (Lang, 1997; Garland, Jones, and Kolodny, 1965).

The Denver Mother's and Children's Project was designed as an early intervention to teach mothering skills and monitor the progress of children. The parent group format of two and a half hours per week provided education on childhood development, opportunities for directed play, role-modelling, and parent discussion groups with a particular focus on parenting and personal issues. The parent discussion group agenda was formulated by the members and subgrouping/networking outside the group was encouraged. The networking was seen as an important outcome of group effectiveness, although it was not measured (Waldo et al., 1987).

The Denver Mother's and Children's Project was very deliberate about admission criteria and the match between the participants and the purpose of the program. The success of the program was based on the participation of the mothers; the involvement of the volunteers and meeting their program goals; the number of children placed in foster care; observations of improved interactions between the mother and child; rehospitalization; success in teaching skills; and the effective use of informal resources. No measures existed to distinguish the efficacy of the group intervention from the program effectiveness. There appears to be some additional sensitivity evident in the attention given to transition times spanning different activities, where transition is typically an anxious time for these parents (Waldo et al., 1987). Responsiveness to these transitions appears to indicate an awareness of individual and group needs and dynamics; however, the program seemed to respond to the anxiety out of a need for things to run smoothly versus using the anxiety and time as an opportunity for group problem solving.

The project also focused on issues related to external pressures and the potential impact these forces might have on the group. Court referrals to the group for the purpose of establishing parent incompetence was a pressure that may have threatened the level of trust between clients and volunteer staff and could have potentially isolated these clients from sources of help. The second main pressure came from those who had the need to see the group as a treatment for schizophrenia. This alternative expectation also could have changed the focus of the group by minimising the purpose of teaching mothering skills and monitoring children as an early intervention project. Introducing these variables as potential threats to the integrity of the program demonstrates our society's desperate need for answers to complex questions regarding the parenting capacities of parents with schizophrenia and a cure-all for schizophrenia. It also informs others of external pressures not often accounted for in these planned interventions (Waldo et al., 1987).

The Threshold Psychosocial Program was designed with an educational focus and a group format to assist in the formation of a safe, secure, nonjudgemental peer group. A mothers' therapy group, a child development class, a stress management component, a health issues focus, and a parenting skills group formed the spectrum of group interventions. This was a comparative study where clients were randomly assigned to a home visiting program, the psychosocial program, or a control group. Effectiveness measures included rehospitalisation, member satisfaction, living independently, and pursuing life goals, i.e., employment. The outcome of this program indicated the treatment programs had a greater effect than the control group; however, data were not provided to validate this claim (Dincin et al., 1995; Zeitz, 1995).

Cohler, Stott, and Musik (1996) compared the efficacy of a Home Care Program (no group, a weekly home visit program of support, parenting focus, and case management), with the Thresholds Program (group-based, intensive, four-day-per-week program). They found there were no significant differences in outcomes between the two approaches in spite of the intensity of the Thresholds Program. All parents showed improvement in social rehabilitation. The group format enabled some mothers to absorb and apply new knowledge about their children's development and the educational groups appeared to have an impact on self-esteem based on improved learning. They also report that the group format provided opportunities for relating to other adults that appeared to reduce the amount of social isolation. Although the literature speaks extensively about the isolation of those with schizophrenia, it does not appear, in this analysis, as an extraneous or confounding variable that had an impact on the effect in either study.

The PACT Program, as described by Goodman and Brumley (1990) of Emory University, was designed as a group intervention with the purpose of developing parent skills using a format of weekly, two-hour meetings over a nine-month time frame. They also refer to the model as a parent support group but give no information about the support aspect. They provide an account of the group structure and content but do not provide any data about the efficacy of this group intervention.

Goodman (1984) also describes the PACE Program run in the Bronx area of New York. Mothers attend an "entry group" designed as a weekly education and discussion group intended as a forum to minimise fears and to provide information for assessment. Following several months of "entry group," mothers are transferred, two at a time, to the "core group." The core group is a five-hour-per-day, four-day-per-week format that includes psychotherapy, competence training, social and recreational groups, cultural activities, and informal opportunities. The core group's success is measured by the growth of the network, "when [the] group begins to function as a supportive network" (p. 68). This speaks of a group functioning as an autonomous, cohesive entity (Lang, 1997). This frame of reference appears congruent with the roles and tasks assigned to the group leaders in the project: bonding with the individual members, facilitating group growth, and eventually helping members terminate. "In time the group begins to take on a life of its own" (Goodman, 1984, p. 68). It is at this point in time, when the group takes on a life of its own, that the group worker begins to withdraw from the membership of the group.

The group is used as a medium to transfer dependence, initially focussed on a staff person in the entry phase, to interdependence on informal networks established in the group process. Those requiring a level of structure and support after the core group can move to an open-ended, task-oriented group conducted by a staff member. This group is also used as a crisis support for those who are discharged from the program. No data are available to address the efficacy of this approach; however, the process described is an indicator itself of a level of success achieved by those mothers who developed their own supportive networks independent of format resources.

Lucas et al. (1984) researched the effect of a child group and two parent groups: one direct counselling group based on social learning theory and a second parent education group based on cognitive skill building. Outcome measures were conducted only on the child group participants. The study indicated an improvement in the children as the intervention proceeded.

Lyons-Ruth, Botein, and Grunebaum (1984) based their intervention on "experience [that] had established the value of groups for mothers of young children" (p. 110). They compared the efficacy of a group approach with a home visit program. The account of the group intervention speaks about an elongated process of working with individuals in their homes and gradually introducing the concept of group intervention. To allay fears and apprehensions of scapegoating in meetings, the worker destigmatised the concept through a patient, long-term transition into a group modality. Group leaders promoted norms of social equality among members and tolerance for noncommittal participation. This usually entailed a three- to four-month period of inconsistent attendance that tested the reliability of the leader before a secure alliance was formed. This group could be described as a transitional group (Lang, 1997) because the purpose, commitment, and acceptance of the group was being tested by individual members over an extended period.

Lyons-Ruth, Botein, and Grunebaum (1984) describe the group as it moves to an autonomous entity: "highly cohesive groups coalesced which remained stable for a period of several years" (p. 112). The group process offered correction, nurturance, problem solving, and the creation of helpful networks outside the group. The group worker role at this stage is described as helping the group regulate anger, tension, and depression, which allowed for a greater depth of intimacy; however, details of how the group worker accomplished this task were not available.

The efficacy of the home visit program and the group intervention is cited anecdotally. There was no difference found between the two programs. Lyons-Ruth, Botein, and Grunebaum (1984) found that not all mothers would agree to participate in a group. In this study, only 64 percent of the eligible participants agreed to attend group. They also found that home visits combined with the group format were critical in maintaining high rates of participation.

Nikkel (1994) cautioned against the singular use of group education formats because persons with serious mental illness may not be able to generalise the material; therefore, individual attention is necessary in conjunction with the group modality. Nikkel's study indicated that group therapy provides a forum for discussing relationship skills and fosters the building of networks. No data were available to support his claims or the efficacy of group interventions. Many other programs are cited in the literature, such as the Henderson Hospital program where all treatment is group based and the group per se functions as a microcosm of society. The focus at Henderson Hospital is on interpersonal interactions. Case examples provide a qualitative perspective, but analysis and efficacy data were not included (Norton and Dolan, 1996). The St. Louis model (Whitman and Accardo, 1989) used unobtrusive modelling as strategy within the group modality and "found that parents enjoyed and benefited from group as well as from more individual sessions" (p. 247). Rogosch, Mowbray, and Bogat (1992) report that emotional support from network members influenced self-esteem, which predicted more adaptive parenting attitudes, and that chronicity and severity of schizophrenia predicted less adaptive parenting attitudes. These accounts speak of group intervention efforts that provide some anecdotal reports of success.

In addition, many other authors, speaking from a standpoint of practise wisdom, promote the use of a group modality (Gross, Fogg, and Tucker, 1995). Seeman (1996) indicates that "parenting classes or groups are an important adjunct to the mothers suffering from schizophrenia" (p. 192) and that, furthermore, "impairments . . . may be improved by specific pharmacotherapy, by parenting groups, by psychotherapy support or by cognitive-behavioral techniques" (p. 195). At the same time, Seeman cautions against the use of group intervention for those individuals who experience increased anxiety with social stimulation.

Waldo et al. (1987) comment that "parenting groups where such common parental fears can be aired and strategies of intervention discussed and practiced are of particular value to psychosis-prone parents" (p. 196). Nicholson and Blanch (1994) support the notion of a peer support/discussion group for parents as part of the rehabilitation process, indicating that a forum for discussing fears and concerns as well as sharing specific coping strategies is critical.

Benton and Schroeder (1990) and Penn and Meuser (1996) are somewhat more cautious in their willingness to support the efficacy of group interventions. Benton and Schroeder's meta-analysis of twenty-seven studies regarding social skills training for individuals with schizophrenia in the context of a group modality revealed that social behavior improved when behavioral measures were applied. They imply that a very narrow focus of measurement may be restrictive in providing a broader perspective of improvement. This may include the generalisability of skills as well as attitudinal changes that are important from a parenting perspective. Penn and Meuser (1996) indicate that more controlled group trials are needed; "work needs to be conducted to determine the key components of group social skills training" (p. 609).

Ahmed and Goldman (1994), in their study of cognitive rehabilitation using a group model, demonstrated empirically an improvement in communication and social skills. Qualitative improvement in group behavior and cognitive processing skills was noted as well as a positive experience by members' ratings of the group's effectiveness. The group intervention, however, did not provide a reduction of psychiatric symptoms. Process learning was evident as members were able to improve their social interaction by learning to become aware of the rules in the communication process.

This collection of literature provides an array of responses to the efficacy of group interventions specific to parents with a serious mental illness. The review raises questions, stimulates ideas, and creates a context for further discussion. The next section discusses the implications of this information.

IMPLICATIONS

The absence of qualitative and quantitative data is reflective of the attention given to this topic to date. The absence of data, however, may be an indicator of changing times versus an issue of oversight or neglect. Values of previous generations promoted involvement of the extended family as a response to mental illness. On the other hand, values of previous generations also sent individuals with serious mental illness to institutions and adopted away the children if they were not cared for by relatives. The values of society today promote less institutionalisation, more community ownership, and helping strategies that protect the rights of all—including the right of a seriously mentally ill person to parent. These changing values have brought the issues of parenting with impairments to the forefront. In response, social service networks have attempted to accommodate in a trial and error manner. The group intervention strategies for seriously mentally ill parents are a recent trend in the literature. The majority of literature written on the subject emanates from the 1980s and continues to the present.

The experience of practise has presently gained sufficient proportion to point researchers in the direction of developing an empirical base of evidence. One indicator of support to move in this direction comes from a thrust to incorporate policy into mental health legislation. Nicholson (1995) and Blanch, Nicholson, and Purcell (1994) conducted a survey of U.S. states and the District of Columbia and found that only sixteen states collected data on whether women who receive public sector services have young children. Four states have residential programs for mentally ill women and their children and approximately 50 percent of the states have programs for assessing parenting skills and outpatient services focussed on improving skills. The publicising of deficits in social programs and policy such as this will provide some impetus to incorporate inclusive policies for this population.

It also appears from this review that group interventions are a necessary part of a comprehensive treatment plan for seriously mentally ill parents. To take a step back, however, points to an inherent assumption that seriously mentally ill parents require a group intervention to combat isolation and enhance social networks. In the study by Lyons-Ruth, Botein, and Grunebaum (1984), the acceptance rate for group intervention was 64 percent. In another study by Dixon and Lehman (1995) on group interventions with families, only six out of eleven families agreed to participate. Perhaps this is an indication that a significant proportion of seriously mentally ill individuals prefer forms of intervention other than the group. This may also be an indication of preferences for interventions that provide less social stimulation or perhaps the need for preparation and readiness to engage in a group format. It may be counterindicated to include individuals who were socialised in a family context that favors a secluded lifestyle, a small number of friends, and individualised activities in a group context that is socially intense, intimate, or involving a high degree of interpersonal process.

In practise, it may be more appropriate to provide a range of options which includes groups that are less socially stimulating and more task or interest focused. Building in choice is one step towards creating a safe context between the worker and the group members. Low expectations regarding group commitment, minimal requirements for participation and attendance, and a focus on reinforcing individual strengths and competencies are features of a "broad range model" (Lang, 1997) promoting engagement of individuals into a group format. Practise possibilities include the development of assessment tools, the enhancement of a broad range model, and educational promotion of group benefits.

Assessment tools to accurately determine treatment preferences and group readiness may help to channel parents into treatment modalities best suited for them and accepted by them versus using a trial and error approach with assumed universal efficacy. Understanding the lifestyle of individuals through an assessment function will help to determine the potential or role of a group format. Interest inventories, strength inventories, individual aspirations, and levels of social interactions and needs are a few categories that an assessment could uncover in the process of determining the appropriateness and readiness for a group intervention. Matching an individual to an appropriate group context may enhance the success of a group intervention.

Development of the broad range model, articulated by Lang (1997), can contribute to a continuum of understanding regarding groups that may be more responsive to the needs of this parent population. A number of studies indicated group interventions that spanned several years. These groups did not start with intense structure or content but rather developed their cohesive dynamics and increased support over time. In this sense, the genesis of such a group was comparatively unique to the looks and behaviors of a democratically functioning entity as described earlier in this chapter.

Development of a broad range model can provide new insight and specific strategies into responses for the seriously mentally ill parent, and especially for those individuals who are not ready for an intense group experience. My contact and interactions with such a group confirmed the need to move at the group's pace and with the group's agenda. A walking trip to the nearby market to review nutritional aspects of menu planning for children is an example of a natural, non-threatening opportunity to develop common experiences on the road to cohesion and group support. The implications of this type of group activity within the context of a psychiatric facility, however, are significant.

It is difficult for institutions and staff to rationalise this type of semistructured activity as a therapeutic response and, even more difficult, to have it recognised as a legitimate form of intervention with this population. The clear articulation of a model and subsequent research to validate the use of such a model is missing. Similarly, the studies cited in this chapter did not provide empirical evidence supporting the types of group formats, contents, and structures that best serve the needs of this population. Intuitively, there is an experiential knowledge that these interventions work but empirically there is no evidence; therefore, it is that much harder to persuade and convince organisations and colleagues that there is efficacy in group interventions and specifically in a broad range approach.

Education about groups for the seriously mentally ill is another consideration for practise. If individuals are going to make decisions about the type of services they will use, they need to know more about group interventions as an option. Information and discussion sessions about group formats are one way to assist those parents with serious mental illness to make informed decisions. Providing this education as another application of group intervention may also begin to demonstrate to participants the various benefits of the group structure.

Continuing to provide updates within our working environments and informing organizations and colleagues about the advantages and efficacy of group interventions is another practical approach to enhancing support and openness to group interventions. There is a public relations function for group workers to consider as part of our educational tasks. Developing awareness among our colleagues and within our agencies is an effective way of building momentum and support for continuing social work with group efforts.

From another perspective, many of the articles are about mothers and their children as opposed to fathers and their children or parents and their children. No statistics are available on the prevalence of single mothers with a serious mental illness who have children in their care in comparison to single fathers with a serious mental illness with children in their care or even dual parent families with one or both parents with a serious mental illness with children. It may be that prevalence rates are associated with the concentration of studies on mothers. Contributing to this may be our societal attitudes that continue to place the burden of child rearing responsibility on the mother. In spite of unknown demographics, this situation begs the question "Where are the fathers and what supportive roles and responsibilities are they able to contribute to parenting?" Consideration of potential involvement of the fathers may also alleviate some of the demand on format services. As practitioners, we can explore avenues to involve the fathers and ask for their involvement in the process of planning for their children.

The issue of confidentiality was skirted in many of the articles in this review yet it has a tremendous potential for negative impact on the implementation of a group intervention. Child welfare legislation (Child and Family Services Act, 1984) in Ontario (Ministry of the Attorney General, Toronto) has very stringent criteria regarding children at risk. The stigma associated with mental illness, the practical realities of impairments related to serious mental illness, the lack of policy to guide decisions regarding parenting responsibilities of the seriously mentally ill, and the lack of resources to respond to these unique parenting needs weigh heavily in favour of the apprehension of the children. The concept of a group as a nurturing and safe place to disclose about parenting practise and issues places the group workers in a position of breaching confidentiality. Given the legislation regarding children at risk, professionals are bound by duty to report such events. The group worker is in a precarious position of losing the nurturing, safe environment and the trust of the group, and the group member is placed in the vulnerable situation of losing his or her children.

From a practise perspective, the limitations of the law restrict the type of structure and content available in a group intervention and therefore limit the possibilities for these parents. What may be helpful in the province of Ontario is a strong liaison between the services providing group interventions for parents with serious mental illness and the child welfare agencies responsible for the protection of children. Group workers can advocate on behalf of these parents for a greater acceptance of creative alternatives to support the seriously mentally ill parent and his or her child at whatever level of parenting capacity he or she is functioning. Helping sustain the parent-child relationship and, at the same time, ensuring the protection of children, is a concern for the parent, the child welfare system, and the group worker providing a service. Other alternatives, such as specialised support groups for parents, a foster parent system that promotes parents visiting in the foster home, an intensive group intervention within high-risk neighborhoods, or funding for child care to give parents a break, may be solutions for parents and the welfare authorities.

Developing social action groups with these parents to effect change in legislation or lobby for resources may be another response for group worker involvement. In cases where children have already been apprehended, there may be a group worker role in bringing the parties together. The group worker function in this context would be to mediate a reasonable decision for both parties.

The development of contingency plans with individuals prior to a group experience may alleviate a crisis for the group worker and the member in the event of a disclosure. These plans may involve extended family members, friends, or other community resources that become a network of support for the seriously mentally ill parent. Development of contingency plans with the group may be another option to respond to crisis as a result of disclosure. Involvement or informing authorities of contingencies may serve to minimise the tension between parents and authorities and perhaps develop a greater appreciation and acceptance of alternatives with the authorities.

The idea of a consumer-based approach for medically oriented services is a relatively new concept. Asking parents what they think is important in their treatment, and supportive intervention is not a well-developed theme in the literature reviewed. Nicholson et al. (1993) and Nicholson (1995) have spearheaded a consumer-based program of research for parents with psychiatric disabilities and their families. The use of focus groups has provided data that begin to address the scope of the problem from a parent's perspective. "Consumer input answers the relevance of questions asked, the sensitivity of procedures and usefulness of answers" (Nicholson, 1995, p. 9). Future efforts on behalf of parents with serious mental illnesses will be better integrated with the inclusion of input from participants.

This is not a new concept for social work with groups. The implication for practise, in a medical model, is to buffer the influence of the pathological views with a focus on group work values. It is also our task to promote and validate group work values, principles, and effectiveness with our colleagues through our writings, publications, and research efforts.

Social work with groups goes beyond participation in a group modality. Practise includes promotion and research. Clarity of models, articulation of the values and principles supporting social work with groups, a belief and commitment to these core tenets, experience to reinforce our knowledge and beliefs, and quality research to validate our group interventions is the recipe to move forward with social work with groups. Application of this recipe begins with each of us as group workers.

CONCLUSION

The population of parents with serious mental illness has very unique challenges to overcome. They are hampered with disabilities that affect them individually and have an impact on their partnerships, families, and communities. The support offered to assist with these circumstances has often included a group intervention. The use of groups appears to have achieved a level of success; however, the empirical evidence to support these claims is waning. There is a continuing need for interventions and responses for parents with serious mental illness in helping them cope with the duties of parenthood. There is also a continuing need to validate these efforts, beyond anecdotal accounts, with empirical data.

Acknowledging and supporting the needs of parents and children alike may be accomplished at a number of levels. Involvement at the macro level through research specific to the efficacy of group interventions will identify strategies that will be most useful to parents. Advocating for policy change that considers the impairment of parents with serious mental illness will help to channel resources to these populations. The integration of creative alternatives, supportive communities, and working relationships between service providers and child welfare agencies will begin to enhance and consolidate services at the mezzo level. Fostering consumer-based strategies at the micro level will support the strengths of participants and promote a level of control over their impairments. These actions will begin to address the needs of parents with a serious mental illness.

As I interpret social work with groups in its broadest context it includes the ability to respond and be effective at a variety of levels including theoretical development, assessment, broad range group work, advocacy, mediation, research, and publication. To move forward as a legitimate and recognised intervention, social work with groups must incorporate each of these levels into a conceptual base and must develop each of these levels with purpose and proactive planning. Lee (1986) quotes Middleman, who leaves a challenge for us to consider as we go about our group work activities: "Group work is for all social workers to use according to what needs to be done rather than what they feel comfortable doing" (Middleman, 1978, p. 16).

REFERENCES

Ahmed, M. and Goldman, J. (1994). Cognitive rehabilitation of adults with severe and persistent mental illness: A group model. *Community Mental Health Journal*, 30(4), 385-394.

Bachrach, L. and Nadelson, C. (Eds.) (1988). *Treating Chronically Mentally Ill Women*. Washington, DC: American Psychiatric Press.

Benton, M. and Schroeder, H. (1990). Social skills training with schizophrenics: A meta-analytic evaluation. *Journal of Consulting and Clinical Psychology*, 58(6), 741-747.

Blanch, A., Nicholson, J., and Purcell, J. (1994). Parents with severe mental illness and their children: The need for human service integration. *The Journal of Mental Health Administration*, 21(4), 388-396.

Breton, M. (1985). Reaching and engaging people, issues and practice principles. *Social Work with Groups*, 8(3), 7-21.

Cohler, B., Stott, F., and Musik, J. (1996). Distressed parents and their young children: Interventions for families at risk. In Gopfert, M., Webster, J., and Seeman, M. (Eds.), *Parental Psychiatric Disorder: Distressed Parents and Their Families*. Cambridge: Cambridge University Press.

Cook, J. and Cohler, B. (1986). Reciprocal socialisation and the care of offspring with cancer and with schizophrenia. In Datan, N., Greene, A., and Reese, H. (Eds.), *Life-Span Developmental Psychology: Intergenerational Relations*. Hillsdale, NJ: Lawrence Erlbaum Associates.

Coverdale, J. and Aruffo, J. (1989). Family planning needs of female chronic psychiatric outpatients. *American Journal of Psychiatry*, 146(11), 1489-1491.

Dincin, J., Zeitz, M., Farrell, D., Harrington, L., Green, W., Pavick, D., Rucks, C., and Illing, P. (1995). Special programs for special groups. *New Directions for Mental Health Services*, 68, 55-73.

Dixon, L. and Lehman, A. (1995). Family intervention for schizophrenia. *Schizophrenia Bulletin,* 21(4), 631-643.

Dunn, B. (1993). Growing up with a psychiatric mother: A retrospective study. *American Orthopsychiatric,* 63(2), 177-189.

Falck, H. (1995). Central characteristics of social work with groups: A sociocultural analysis. In Kurland, R. and Salmon, R. (Eds.), *Group Work Practice in a Troubled Society.* Binghamton, NY: The Haworth Press.

Field, T., Healy, B., and Goldstein, S. (1988). Infants of depressed mothers show "depressed" behavior even with non-depressed adults. *Child Development,* 26, 40-50.

Gangbar, R. (1997). Mental illness and the family. Presentation, April 16. The Clarke Institute of Psychiatry, Toronto, Ontario.

Garland, J., Jones, H., and Kolodny, R. (1965). A model for stages of development in social work groups. In Bernstein, S. (Ed.) (1973), *Explorations in Group Work.* Boston: Milford House.

Garvin, C. (1992). A task centered group approach to work with the chronically mentally ill. *Social Work with Groups,* 15(2/3), 67-80.

Garvin, C. (1997). *Contemporary Group Work,* Third Edition. Boston: Allyn and Bacon.

Germain, C. and Gitterman, A. (1980). *The Life Model of Social Work Practice.* New York: Columbia University Press.

Gidron, B., Gutterman, N., and Hartman, H. (1990). Stress and coping patterns of participants and non-participants in self-help groups for parents of the mentally ill. *Community Mental Health Journal,* 26, 483-496.

Gitterman, A. (1986). The reciprocal model: A change in the paradigm. *Social Work with Groups,* 8(4), 29-37.

Goodman, C. (1984). The Pace Family Treatment and Education Program: A public health approach to parental competence and promotion of mental health. In Cohler, B. and Musik, J. (Eds.), *Intervention Among Psychiatrically Impaired Parents and Their Young Children.* San Francisco: Jossey-Bass.

Goodman, S. and Brumley, E. (1990). Schizophrenic and depressed mothers: Relational deficits in parenting. *Developmental Psychology,* 26(1), 31-39.

Gopfert, M., Webster, J., and Seeman, M. (Eds.) (1996). *Parental Psychiatric Disorder: Distressed Parents and Their Families.* Cambridge: Cambridge University Press.

Gottesman, I. (1991). *Schizophrenia Genesis.* New York: Freeman.

Gross, D., Fogg, L., and Tucker, S. (1995). The efficacy of parent training for promoting positive parent-toddler relationships. *Research in Nursing and Health,* 18, 489-499.

Halgin, R. and Whitbourne, S. (1993). *Abnormal Psychology.* Fort Worth: Harcourt Brace Jovanovich College Publishers.

Hamilton, E., Jones, M., and Hammon, C. (1993). Maternal interaction style in affected disordered, physically disabled and normal women. *Family Process,* 32(3), 329-340.

Hogarty, G., Anderson, C., Reiss, D., Kornblith, S., Greenwald, D., Javna, C., and Madonia, M. (1986). Family psychoeducation, social skills training, and maintenance chemotherapy in the aftercare treatment of schizophrenia. *Archives of General Psychiatry,* 43, 633-642.

Jenkins, A. (1996). NEWPIN: A creative mental health service for parents and children. In Cohler, B. and Musik, J. (Eds.), *Intervention Among Psychiatrically Impaired Parents and Their Young Children.* San Francisco: Jossey-Bass.

Kanas, N. (1991). Group therapy with schizophrenic patients: A short-term, homogeneous approach. *International Journal of Group Psychotherapy,* 41(1), 33-47.

Kane, C., DiMartino, E., and Jiminez, M. (1990). A comparison of short-term psychoeducational and support groups for relatives coping with chronic schizophrenia. *Archives of Psychiatric Nursing,* 6, 343-353.

Kassis, J., Boothroyd, P., and Ben-Dror, R. (1990). The family support group: Families and Professionals in Partnership. *Psychosocial Rehabilitation Journal,* 13, 92-96.

Kurland, R. and Salmon, R. (1996). Making joyful noise: Presenting, promoting, and portraying group work to and for the profession. In Stempler, B., Glass, M., and Savinelli, C. (Eds.), *Social Group Work Today and Tomorrow.* Binghamton, NY: The Haworth Press.

Lang, N. (1997). University of Toronto, Faculty of Social Work. SWK 4602 Course Syllabus. Spring.

Lee, J. (1986). Seeing it whole: Social work with groups within an integrative perspective. *Social Work with Groups,* 8(4), 39-50.

Leff, J., Shavit, N., Strachan, A., Glass, L., and Vaughn, C. (1989). A trial of family therapy. A relatives group for schizophrenia. *British Journal of Psychiatry,* 154, 58-66.

Lucas, L., Montgomery, S., Richardson, D., and Rivers, P. (1984). Reducing the risk of mental illness to children of distressed mothers. In Cohler, B. and Musik, J. (Eds.), *Intervention Among Psychiatrically Impaired Parents and Their Young Children.* San Francisco: Jossey-Bass.

Lyons-Ruth, K., Botein, S., and Grunebaum, H. (1984). Reaching the hard-to-reach: Serving isolated and depressed mothers with infants in the community. In Cohler, B. and Musik, J. (Eds.), *Intervention Among Psychiatrically Impaired Parents and Their Young Children.* San Francisco: Jossey-Bass.

McNamee, J., Lipman, E., and Hicks, F. (1995). A single mothers' group for mothers of children attending an outpatient psychiatric clinic: Preliminary results. *Canadian Journal of Psychiatry,* 40, 383-388.

Middleman, R. (1978). Returning group process to group work. *Social Work with Groups,* 1(1), 15-26.

Middleman, R. and Wood, G. (1995). Contextual group work: Apprehending the elusive obvious. In Kurland, R. and Salmon, R. (Eds.), *Group Work Practice in a Troubled Society*. Binghamton, NY: The Haworth Press.

Mowbray, C., Oyserman, D., Zemencuk, J., and Ross, S. (1995). Motherhood for women with serious mental illness: Pregnancy, childbirth, and the postpartum period. *American Orthopsychiatric Association, Inc.*, 65(1), 21-38.

Nadelson, C. (1996). Foreword. In Cohler, B. and Musik, J. (Eds), *Among Psychiatrically Impaired Parents and Their Young Children*. San Francisco: Jossey-Bass.

Nicholson, J. (1995). Parents with psychiatric disabilities and their families: A consumer-based program of research. *Community Support Network News*, 10(3). Boston: Center for Psychiatric Rehabilitation.

Nicholson, J. and Blanch, A. (1994). Rehabilitation for parenting roles for people with serious mental illness. *Psychosocial Rehabilitation Journal*, 18(1), 109-119.

Nicholson, J., Geller, J., Fisher, W., and Dion, G. (1993). State policies and programs that address the needs of mentally ill mothers in the public sector. *Hospital and Community Psychiatry*, 44(5), 484-489.

Nikkel, R. (1994). Areas of skill training for persons with mental illness and substance use disorders: Building skills for successful community living. *Community Mental Health Journal*, 30, 61-72.

Norton, K. and Dolan, B. (1996). Personality disorder and parenting. In Gopfert, M., Webster, J., and Seeman, M. (Eds.), *Parental Psychiatric Disorder: Distressed Parents and Their Families*. Cambridge: Cambridge University Press.

Papell, C. (1992). Group work with new populations: Knowledge and knowing. *Social Work with Groups*, 15(2/3), 23-36.

Penn, D. and Meuser, K. (1996). Research update on the psychosocial treatment of schizophrenia. *American Journal of Psychiatry*, 153(5), 607-617.

Pound, A. (1996). Parental affective disorder and childhood disturbance. In Gopfert, M., Webster, J., and Seeman, M. (Eds.), *Parental Psychiatric Disorder: Distressed Parents and Their Families*. Cambridge: Cambridge University Press.

Rogosch, F., Mowbray, C., and Bogat, A. (1992). Determinants of parenting attitudes in mothers with severe psychopathology. *Development and Psychopathology*, 4(3), 469-487.

Rubovits, P. (1996). Project CHILD: An intervention programme for psychotic mothers and their young children. In Gopfert, M., Webster, J., and Seeman, M. (Eds.), *Parental Psychiatric Disorder: Distressed Parents and Their Families*. Cambridge: Cambridge University Press.

Schwartz, W. (1961). The social worker in the group. In *New Perspectives on Services to Groups* (p. 13). New York: National Association of Social Workers.

Schwartz, W. (1986). The group work tradition and social work practice. *Social Work with Groups*, 8(4), 7-27.

Seeman, M. (1996). The mother with schizophrenia. In Gopfert, M., Webster, J., and Seeman, M. (Eds.), *Parental Psychiatric Disorder: Distressed Parents and Their Families*. Cambridge: Cambridge University Press.

Waldo, M., Roath, M., Levine, W., and Freedman, R. (1987). A model program to teach parenting skills to schizophrenic mothers. *Hospital and Community Psychiatry,* 38(10), 1110-1112.

Walsh, J. (1987). The family education and support group: A psychoeducational aftercare program. *Psychosocial Rehabilitation Journal,* 10, 51-61.

Wang, A. and Goldschmidt, V. (1994). Interviews of psychiatric inpatients about their family situation and young children. *Acta Psychiatrica Scandinavia,* 90, 459-465.

Weintraub, S. (1987). Risk factors in schizophrenia: The Stony Brook high risk project. *Schizophrenia Bulletin,* 13(3), 439-450.

Whitman, B. and Accardo, P. (1989). *When a Parent Is Mentally Retarded.* Baltimore: Paul Brookes.

Zeitz, M. (1995). The mothers' project: A clinical case management system. *Articles,* 19(1), 55-62.

Zemencuk, J., Rogosch, F., and Mowbray, C. (1995). The seriously mentally ill women in the role of the parent: Characteristics, parenting sensitivity, and needs. *Psychosocial Rehabilitation Journal,* 18(3), 77-92.

Chapter 11

Post–Legal Adoption Treatment Groups: Intervening with Families Who Experience Failed Adoptions

Karen V. Harper-Dorton

INTRODUCTION

The challenge to reduce the risk of broken attachments and failed relationships between parents and an adopted child calls not only for understanding the risks involved but also for their prevention and treatment. Numerous studies document increased numbers of children returning to temporary care after adoption disruption, particularly among families who adopt older children and other special needs children (Westhus and Cohen, 1990). The study reported here involves researchers and agency-based treatment staff working together to (1) identify families likely to experience adoption disruption, (2) provide post–legal adoption treatment with groups of children and parents, and (3) report success rates among families from these treatment groups. This project was funded by the Department of Health and Human Services to develop post–legal adoption group treatment services to families at risk of adoption disruption. Assisted by agency-based adoption professionals, the authors (Harper and Loadman, 1992) developed a predictive model of adoption disruption, helped develop curricula for parents and children in post–legal adoption counseling groups for families at risk of adoption dissolu-

Supported by DHHS, ACF Funding, this demonstration project was cosponsored with Lucas County Children Services and Jewish Family Services, Toledo, Ohio, in association with Dr. Karen V. Harper-Dorton and Dr. William E. Loadman, principal researchers.

tion, directed agency-based practitioners in conducting post–legal adoption treatment groups, and evaluated outcomes of this group intervention.

Presented in this report are findings from a two-year project predicting adoptive families at risk of adoption disruption from a study involving 219 families with finalized adoptions, forty families who self-identified as needing post–legal adoption treatment services, and forty-nine families in the process of adoption finalizations. The forty families threatened with adoption disruption were identified as seeking treatment at a point where they were considering returning their adopted children to the child welfare agency.

Group intervention was selected as the model of choice for intervening with adopted children and their parents at risk of ending their adoptions and terminating family relationships due to very troubled and emotionally damaging family dynamics. Working with these families in groups provided a medium for communication, an opportunity for sharing experiences with peer families, and, most important, the opportunity for adopted children to meet and share their experiences with other adoptees. Curricula for post–legal adoption treatment groups with adopted children and their parents will be shared along with participant feedback and brief outcome findings.

ADOPTION DISRUPTION/DISSOLUTION: DEFINITIONS AND OVERVIEW

Terminated adoptive placements are "disruptions" that occur before finalization; dissolutions occur only after adoptions are finalized. Terminations after adoption finalization result in dissolved adoptions that involve returning a child to an agency. The lack of distinction between disrupted and dissolved adoptions is not only true for children but is true for much of the research in the field of adoptions. Disruption is commonly used in much of the literature to include phenomena of both dissolution and disruption when referring to failed adoptive relationships in the lives of children. For the child, the trauma of lost familial relationships is much the same regardless of the legal status of the placement. For the purpose of this report, families who terminate the adoption or its process will be referred to as disruption regardless of legal status.

Many factors have been associated with adoption disruption. Extensive research by Barth and Berry identifies predictive factors of adoption disruption (Barth and Berry, 1988; Berry and Barth, 1990). Their work identifies five major predictive factors of disruption: a child with a previous adoptive placement, a non–foster adoption, a child with special problems, the placement of a child at an older age, and an adoptive mother with a higher education. Children, parents, and agency-related factors contribute to adoption disruption and can be found throughout the literature. These factors are summarized as follows.

Child factors include a child's older age, an inability to attach to adoptive parents, sibling groups, the child not having a relationship with the adoptive family before the placement, the presence of emotional and behavioral problems, previous multiple placements, and being a child of male gender (Berry and Barth, 1990; Schmidt, Rosenthal, and Bombeck, 1988; Boyne et al., 1984; Partridge, Hornby, and McDonald, 1986).

Parent factors have been determined to include poorly defined roles within the family functioning, infertility, single parents, high expectations for the child, the education level of the mother, personalities with high egocentricism or self-centeredness, and inadequate financial resources (Smith and Sherwen, 1983; LePere, 1987; Barth and Berry, 1988; Bourguignon and Watson, 1989; Zwimpher, 1983).

Agency factors, although not as extensive, include inadequate information concerning the adoptive child and her or his family history and inadequate services that link families with support systems such as parent groups (Barth and Berry, 1988; Rosenthal and Groze, 1990; Nelson, 1985).

The rates of adoption disruption and dissolution are not agreed upon in the literature. Barth and Berry (1988) found that 10 percent of adoptions disrupt. Tremitiere (1979) reported that 10 percent of six- to twelve-year-old children experience disruption but that twelve- to eighteen-year-olds experience a 14 percent disruption rate. In studying "hard-to-place children," Boyne et al. (1984) reported that 23 percent experienced disruption. Over a five-year period, Fein, Davies, and Knight (1979) found that up to 31 percent of adoptions are likely to disrupt. Based on their review of the literature, Westhus and Cohen (1990) concluded that, on average, between 8 and 15 percent of adoptions disrupt. Clearly there is a range of findings and a mix of disrupted and dissolved cases in the studies reported. Nevertheless, the number of children experiencing terminated adoptions warrants further research that can impact program design in the service arena.

DEMOGRAPHICS OF THE POPULATION STUDIED

The population included 219 adoptive families of one county in Ohio. Adoptions in these families became final during the 2-year period preceding this study. There were 193 families whose adoptions remained intact while 26 (11.9 percent) experienced adoption dissolution. Profiles of adoptive parents and children were constructed based on data gathered from agency records.

Adoptive parents' characteristics in this study suggest that mothers and fathers were approximately 40 years of age, were usually racially matched with their child, and that at least 96 percent had not been adopted themselves. Only 19 percent of the parents were related by family origin to their child. Among the parents, 11.9 percent (N = 26) reported having a great deal of information about their child's background, 47.0 percent (N = 103) reported having some information, and 35.2 percent (N = 77) reported having very little information. Of this parent population, 108 (49.3 percent) adopted a child because they wanted to be parents, 55 (25.1 percent) adopted because they wanted a sibling for their birth child in their home, and 34 (15.5 percent) wanted a sibling for an adopted child already in their home. Of the mothers, 79 (42 percent) had completed high school and 70 (38 percent) had at least a partial college education. Among the fathers, 57 (38 percent) had completed high school and 77 (50 percent) had at least some college experience. Thirteen (7 percent) mothers worked part-time and 95 (52 percent) worked full-time.

Adopted children in this population are most often male (N = 117, 53.4 percent). Racial representation includes Caucasian (N = 108, 49.3 percent); African American (N = 75, 34.2 percent); and biracial (N = 10, 4.6 percent). There are 136 (62 percent) living in families with annual incomes of more than $25,000.00. There are 178 (81.3 percent) in subsidized adoptions where financial assistance is provided to help with costs of providing for the child. Among children in this study, 183 (83.6 percent) are reported as having special needs, i.e., either physical, emotional, or mental disabilities; in a sibling group; or past the age of 6 at the time of placement.

Of adopted children in this study, 180 (82.2 percent) are reported to have been abused prior to adoptive placement. Of the adoptive families, 85 (38.8 percent) reported having had the child placed in their care as a foster child before the placement was considered an adoptive placement or adoption legalization occurred. Among the children, 26 (11.8 percent) had experienced at least 1 previous adoptive placement.

THE IMPORTANCE OF POST–LEGAL ADOPTION INTERVENTION

Rearing children and being part of a family is a lifelong process and certainly not one that begins with the placement of a child in need of a permanent family and that ends with happiness forever once the adoption is finalized. Adoptive families, like all families, encounter stresses associated with parenting; experience divorce, separation, deaths, as well as various losses and successes; and often need further professional intervention during the family life cycle. Never has the need for intervention been truer than in today's child welfare arena where children are being placed at older ages and with so many severe and devastating abuse histories. Many of the children available for adoption have special needs, including disabilities, siblings, and previous placements, and they are placed as older children, even as teenagers. Life with children in need of greater nurturance and care often worsens as children grow into their teen years and may display defiant, violent, promiscuous, and other difficult behaviors, sometimes too difficult for families to cope with. The assumption that adoptive families select children to adopt and are selected as desirable families to parent a child in need of a permanent family is outdated in today's world of child rearing.

Partridge, Hornby, and McDonald (1986) call attention to the lack of postplacement services for adoptive families after placement begins. This gap is particularly significant for families who are adopting special needs children or older children. By increasing parental understanding of the child, families may be assisted through the various behavioral problems, the difficult adjustment periods, intense anger and hostility, and the serious self-esteem and attachment difficulties evidenced by some adoptees. Hartman (1984) recognizes the importance of extending postplacement services to adoptive families throughout the years of child rearing. Special needs children in need of families are merely in the process of resolving problems by the time legalization of adoption occurs. Legalization is not a time to close cases for postplacement services.

According to Bourguignon and Watson (1989), critical problem areas among adoptive families are likely to include resolving issues around entitlement to the parents, the claiming of the child into the family, forming new relationships, working with issues of loss and grief, and having different expectations. The resolution of grief and loss associated with adoption is a lifelong need for some adoptees (Goodman and Keefer, 1990). These problem areas frequently contribute to crises that bring families to agencies in search of assistance. As these problems are exacerbated during teenage years, families may seek post–legal adoption services long after finalization. Post–legal adoption services are reported as generally including several information tasks, such as helping families understand adoption, resolve coping, define family identity, and develop problem-solving skills. Special attention is provided to assist families of mixed origin to understand and adjust in situations of transcultural or transracial adoptions. Finally, post–legal adoption services may be necessary to assist families who did not receive counseling or postplacement services prior to legalization.

The objectives for post–legal adoption services are to aid in preventing disruption, resolve crises, and provide ongoing support to adoptive families. Hopefully, this after-the-fact use of post–legal adoption services can be reduced by greater emphasis upon the needs of families and children at the time they enter the lifelong process of adoption. By planning parent and child selection and intervention when the child becomes available for adoption, it may be possible to prevent adoption disruption/dissolution from marring the child's experience. Prevention of disruption/dissolution is cost-effective both in terms of social welfare expenditures and the quality of life of the nation's children.

GROUP SERVICES

Group intervention is viewed as the method of choice as children and adolescents are able to benefit from sharing experiences, validating their feelings, learning from others, learning that they are not alone, and exploring feelings of loss and grief with others in similar circumstances. Parent groups provide the same opportunities for the adopting parents. Groups of parents and children may occasionally be brought together for special purposes but generally the greatest benefits occur in their separate groups. Self-help groups, both for parents and adoptees, may become lifelong support systems (Parenthesis Family Advocates, 1989).

PROGRAM DESIGN

A treatment series of eight group sessions was developed in the belief that parents and children are truly active participants in preventing their own disruption and in acquiring greater understanding of their relationship. The powerful group medium was selected where members could participate freely and use only that which they believed to be helpful while rejecting information that they considered useless. Information and activities were developed with respect to families with children and families with teens. This post–legal adoption group treatment curriculum was designed to respond to the request by parents for help in preventing the loss of an adoptive child due to nearly irreconcilable difficulties. The curriculum was implemented with four groups of ten families, organized by parents, children eleven and under, and teenagers, including one eighteen-year-old. Groups met in community-based agencies and were led by social workers experienced in working with adoptive families. Groups met weekly for an average of two hours per session. Coleaders were assigned to each set of the eight weekly sessions and remained with the group throughout the treatment period.

CURRICULUM

Children's Group Sessions

1. Who Are We?

    Purpose: Build trust
    Objectives: Introduce group members, identify something about yourself, set group rules, "who sounds alike" exercise, intro-

duce what your mother/father like, things you like, complete a family tree with names or colors

2. My "Me"

Purpose: Learn about oneself and others in the group
Objectives: Discuss the importance of names, share likes and dislikes, talk about what your parents named you and why, make a family shield

3. More About My "Me"

Purpose: Learn about oneself
Objectives: Define yourself through disclosure, make "me" collages, name favorite things

4. My Family and Me

Purpose: Identify things valued in oneself and family
Objectives: Discuss parents' biography of you, share a favorite item, draw a favorite item or thing to do

5. Families and Feelings

Purpose: Explore qualities that connect the child to the family
Objectives: Share about family, fill paper boxes with favorite things, talk about family pride, favorite foods, finish statements such as "Things I like about Mom . . ."

6. More About My Families and Me

Purpose: Explore feelings toward present and previous families
Objectives: Explore commitment, identify communication and better communication, do time machine mirror (How old were you when you were adopted? What do you remember? Draw family, clothes, time of year), talk about feeling of belonging in new family

7. How I Feel About Me

Purpose: Explore self-esteem
Objectives: Signature bingo game (Who got the most signatures? Was it hard or easy? What did you learn?) and share "me" boxes

8. Leaving Some of Us with You/Some of You with Me

Purpose: Provide experience of positive closure
Objectives: Discuss endings, make name tags for yourself and your parents, join parents for pizza party

Teens' Group Sessions

1. Who Are We?

Purpose: Introduce group members
Objectives: Icebreakers for teens to share words describing themselves, completion of "I wish . . ." statements, "I want . . ." statements, "My mother/father is . . ." statements, discuss rules and identify something liked and disliked about the group

2. My "Me"

Purpose: Learn about oneself
Objectives: Explore names, what they mean, importance, nicknames, name changes, famous names, construct family shields

3. The Ways We Talk

Purpose: Explore family communication patterns
Objectives: Pick a partner, meet each other, introduce your partner to the group, role-play parent and teen, discuss within the group what you heard and learned

4. The "Right to Know"

Purpose: Allow for self-disclosure
Objectives: Build rapport, trust, share likes and dislikes, build "me" collages

5. My Family and Me

Purpose: Explore circumstances of adoption
Objectives: Discuss adoption experience with group, what is different about your family, what is taboo, prepare for meeting a birth parent

6. A Birth Parent's Experience

   Purpose: Meet and hear a birth parent
   Objectives: Explore an experience of relinquishment, errors, beliefs, explore one's own response to the presentation of a birth parent

7. How I Feel About Me

   Purpose: Explore self-esteem
   Objectives: Share biographies, demonstrate the IALAC (I am lovable and capable) awareness exercise

8. Leaving Some of Us with You/Taking Some of You with Us

   Purpose: Evaluate the group and share with parents' group
   Objectives: Make group collage, join parents for pizza party

Parents' Group Sessions

1. Why Are We Here?

   Purpose: Introduce group members
   Objectives: Establish group rules, parents complete child's biography

2. The Ways We Talk

   Purpose: Explore alternative styles of communication
   Objectives: Sharing, role-play, being picked, how it feels to "be picked"

3. The "Right to Know"

   Purpose: Explore family communication patterns
   Objectives: Explore adoptive/biological families, advantages and disadvantages of disclosure

4. Why They Do What They Do?

   Purpose: Learn about adoptee's experience
   Objectives: Develop empathy, fantasy exercise about loss of a home that just sinks, child's wishes, "you" wishes

5. A Birth Parent's Experience

   Purpose: Expose adoptive parents to birth parent's feelings

Objectives: Views and feelings through birth parent presenting to the group; share and discuss how well child and birth parents knew one another

6. Committing/Connecting/Claiming

   Purpose: Explore feelings about commitment, entitlement, bonding
   Objectives: Emotional entitlement, claiming, and bonding/attachment; fantasy exercises about the ups and downs one can experience in feelings toward oneself

7. Who Are We?

   Purpose: Understand self-esteem
   Objectives: Identify strengths and skills, explore the ups and downs in developing self-esteem

8. Connecting/Closing

   Purpose: Evaluate the group
   Objectives: Identify strengths and skills gained and needed, share time with children, terminate the group

The group intervention described here is intended to be used with adoptive parents and children who are experiencing difficulties in learning to live together. For some families, great problems in adapting to the demands of different life stages arise as the child matures, particularly so in the early teenage years. Families' problems ranged from difficulties with hostile and violent adopted teenagers to the stresses of living with very troubled and destructive younger adoptees. The wisdom of experienced group leaders and experienced adoption professionals produced a group manual that is filled with effective curricula tools and exercises that catch the interests of children and parents in insightful and heartfelt ways. This manual is an organized and instructional tool that makes groups exciting and wonderful.

The group sessions in this demonstration project are designed in the belief that those parents and children who seek greater understanding of their relationship are truly active participants in preventing their own adoption disruption/dissolution. The information and activities are presented with respect for parents and children. Members are encouraged to participate freely but, ultimately, to use only that which they believe to be helpful and can accept or adapt to their situation. Participants must feel free to reject the elements of the program they consider unhelpful or unacceptable.

OUTCOME AND FOLLOW-UP

Outcome evaluation involved a series of affective distance measurements for participants which involved follow-up to evaluate movement to or away from each other and qualitative measures involving powerful revelations such as "I have never met anyone else who is adopted" and "I can't imagine the emptiness if I came home to a home that had disappeared that day."

Using a grid and applying faces with emotional expressions, including happy, sad, angry, sorry, and uninvolved, family members place one another at the distance they feel together or apart. Sharing these diagrams encourages families to reflect upon the degree of intimacy they are feeling. Themes evolving from this exercise show that (1) initially, families were organized with at least one isolate, generally the adopted child; (2) if paired, the child placed himself or herself with one parent; and (3) by the end of eight sessions, all families had changed affective distances, resulting in closer family units. Even though this evaluative measure has not been standardized or tested, there is a general consensus that through communication and growth in post–legal adoption groups, family distance is reduced among members and children generally see their parents as having more positive affective responses.

Group participant feedback was gathered at the end of each session. Collected data and emergent themes provide responses to such open-ended questions as these: (1) What did you get from the session? (2) How do you feel about it? (3) What would you change?

Parents

- Responses ranged from "very helpful" to "didn't get a lot out of it." Feelings were mixed and several participants reported that they did not think it was "geared to me" or "I thought it would be different."

- Most parents reported that their children got "a lot out of it" and that their children's positive responses motivated them to complete all eight sessions. Families in this group shared that they experienced many difficult times with their adopted child(ren) and that sometimes it was "one day at a time." One family reported that they were not "playing with a full deck" to have adopted an older child, that they care about this child and hope to "make it." Families felt more open and reported improved communication and understanding in the home. In general, feelings were mixed, but overall reports showed some improvement in relationships and communication. Most parents reported that their children had developed greater self-esteem.
- One family reported that they had gained a greater understanding of their own feelings about children and adoption.
- In general, all families reported that communication and concern for each other had improved at home and were stimulated by the group experience.

Adoptees

- The strongest benefit was in meeting other adopted children and learning that other adopted children existed.
- Children reported pleasure at having a special friend and most planned to stay in communication with at least one other adoptee from their group.
- About 60 percent of the children reported the birth mother presentation as positive in that they did not know they were missed.
- Children commonly reported increased attention from adoptive parents and saw this as being positive.

Changes Needed

- Leaders should be more open and give the group more time to just talk.
- More joint sessions need to be held for children and parents to share homework from the groups.
- Various comments about the length and the frequency of the sessions surfaced from working parents.

- The participants expressed a strong desire for the outcome of this effort to result in establishing a community-based support service where ongoing group activities would be available for adoptive families.

CONCLUSIONS

Having families respond with new understanding and changed relationships as a result of group intervention validates the importance of group work in situations of troubled adoptions. Many of these same families have experienced previous counseling and various interventions for adoptive placements with little progress. One-year follow-up indicates that, of the families who were previously identified as being at serious risk of disruption, two participating in post–legal adoption treatment groups disrupted and two remained at great risk. Some families consulted additional treatment resources during the year but the families remained intact.

Clearly, the group medium is preferred over individual or family treatment in cases of threatened disruption in adoptive families. Group intervention is used in a wide variety of programs where the communication between families and children is crucial to their emotional and even physical healing (Dolgin et al., 1997). This curriculum model can easily be replicated. Feedback from families, agencies, group leaders, and students involved in the project enthusiastically support the benefits of the experience.

The nature of the child's development and related issues of identity, trust, autonomy, and validation of adolescents must be addressed by group leaders and can be better managed in the group environment (Innes, 1995). The separation of adoptees in groups for younger children and teenagers is necessary so that age-appropriate content and activities can be applied.

Perhaps the greatest potential limitation of post–legal adoption treatment groups is the level of information the group leader must have about adoptive families and the lifelong concerns of adoptees. Leading a group of adoptive families calls for different information than a biological family treatment group. A second concern is that in small towns and rural areas confidentiality may be difficult to maintain.

The translation of knowledge and practice into empirically based outcome evaluation is especially important in establishing the value of treatment efforts such as this. Replication of this effort is called for and can build upon the present work. Greater partnerships between agencies and universities can produce programs to include experimental design and data collection, including funding to validate and standardize instruments developed for specialized treatment efforts like those used in this project. Community/campus partnerships are needed to support the efforts behind this project and this collaboration is important for future program development and outcome reporting.

REFERENCES

Barth, R. P. and Berry, M. (1988). *Adoption and Disruption: Rates, Risks, Responses.* New York: Aldine de Gruyter.

Barth, R. P. and Berry, M. (1990). Preventing adoption disruption. *Prevention in Human Services,* 9, 205-222.

Berry, M. and Barth, R. P. (1990). A study of disrupted adoptive placements of adolescents. *Child Welfare,* 59, 209-225.

Bourguignon, J. -P. and Watson, K. (1989). *Toward Successful Adoption: A Study of Predictors in Special Needs Placements.* Chicago, IL: Illinois Department of Children and Family Services.

Boyne, J., Denby, L., Kettenring, J. R., and Wheeler, W. (1984). *The Shadow of Success: A Statistical Analysis of Outcomes of Adoption of Hard-To-Place Children.* New Jersey: Westfield.

Dolgin, M. J., Somer, E., Zaidel, N., and Zaizov, R. (1997). A structured group intervention for siblings of children with cancer. *Journal of Child and Adolescent Group Therapy,* 7, 3-18.

Fein, E., Davies, L. J., and Knight, G. (1979). Placement stability in foster care. *Social Work,* 24, 136-157.

Goodman, D. and Keefer, B. (1990). *Themes in Adoption.* Columbus, OH: Parenthesis Family Advocates.

Harper, K. V. and Loadman, W. E. (1992). Adoption disruption/dissolution: A predictive model. In *Discovering the New World of Research and Statistics: A Federal/State Partnership* (pp. 107-131). Proceedings of the 32nd National Workshop of the National Association for Welfare Research and Statistics. Columbus, Ohio, August 1-5.

Hartman, A. (1984). *Post-Placement Services in Adoption.* Washington, DC: Child Welfare League of America.

Innes, M. (1995). Parent-teen connection: Towards a family systems approach to group therapy with young "at-risk" adolescents and their parents. *Journal of Child and Adolescent Group Therapy,* 5, 215-228.

LePere, D. W. (1987). Vulnerability to crises during the life-cycle of the adoptive family. *Journal of Social Work and Human Sexuality,* 6, 73-85.

Nelson, K. A. (1985). *On the Frontier of Adoption: A Study of Special Needs Adoptive Families.* New York: Research Center, Child Welfare League of America.

Parenthesis Family Advocates (1989). *Epilogue Post Adoption Services in Ohio.* Columbus, OH: Ohio Department of Human Services.

Partridge, S., Hornby, H., and McDonald, T. (1986). *Learning from Adoption Disruption: Insights for Practice.* Portland, ME: Human Services Development Institute.

Rosenthal, J. A. and Groze, V. (1990). Special-needs adoption: A study of intact families. *Social Service Review,* 64, 475-505.

Schmidt, D. M., Rosenthal, J. A., and Bombeck, B. (1988). Parents' views on adoption disruption. *Children and Youth Services Review,* 10, 119-130.

Smith, D. W. and Sherwen, L. N. (1983). *Mothers and Their Adopted Children: The Bonding Process.* New York: Tiresias Press.

Tremitiere, B. T. (1979). Adoption of children with special needs: The client-centered approach. *Child Welfare,* 58, 681-685.

Westhus, A. and Cohen, J. S. (1990). Preventing disruption of special-needs adoptions. *Child Welfare,* 59, 141-155.

Zwimpher, D. M. (1983). Indicators of adoption breakdown. *Social Casework,* 64, 169-177.

Index

Page numbers followed by the letter "f" indicate figures.

Abstinence model, alcohol, 31
Acceptance, testing of, 88
Action stage, 28
Active prevention, 84
Addams, Jane, 75, 100
Adlerian therapy group model, 149
Adolescents, and community service, 104, 108
Adopted children, characteristics of, 196-197
Adoption Assistance and Child welfare Act of 1980, 147
Adoption disruption/dissolution, 194-196. See also Post–legal adoption families, group work with
Adoptive parents, characteristics of, 196
Agency factors, adoption disruption, 195
Ahmed, M., 181
Al-Anon, 30
Alcoholics Anonymous (AA), 30
Alcoholism, myths surrounding, 30
Alliances, creation of, 1-2
Anonymity, and teleconferencing focus groups, 116-117
"Arbiter of change," 63
Are partners in permanency planning, Families for Reunification group session ten, 154, 163, 164
Aruffo, J., 170
Asian mothers' support project, research and action, 133-134
cultural isolation, 138-139

Asian mothers' support project, research and action (continued)
focus groups, 137-138
gender roles, 139
North Campus Outreach Project (NCOP), 134-137
programming, 139-140
results, 141-142
structural difficulties, 139
survey and program data, 140-141
and synergy through groups, 142-144
Attitudinal myths, 30
Authority theme, 35-37
Avoidance of the Alcoholic Client syndrome, 29

Badham, B., 57
Barnett, Samuel, 100
Barth, R.P., 195
Bayless, L., 150
Be a family reunion specialist, Families for Reunification group session five, 153, 163
Be a loss expert, Families for Reunification group session four, 153, 163
Be an attachment expert, Families for Reunification group session three, 153, 163
"Beginning where the client is," 90

Bennis, W.G., 37
Benton, M., 181
Bereavement support, 116, 118
Berkow, D.N., 82
Berry, M., 195
Bio, W.R., 37, 41
Birth parent self-assessment, 147-149
   Families for Reunification: Partners
      in the Plan, 152-164
   MAPP/GPS, development of,
      149-152
"Blaming the victims," 20
Blanch, A., 180, 189
Bogat, A., 180
Bollinger, D., 9
Botein, S., 179, 182
Bourguignon, J.-P., 198
Boyne, J., 195
Brain death, 118
"Breach of trust," 85
Breton, M., 173
Broad range model, 183
Brown, A., 56
Brownstein, C., 63
Brumley, E., 178
Burrus, S., 104
Bystanders, group members acting as,
   55

Can meet my own needs, Families for
   Reunification group session
   seven, 153, 163, 164
Career factors, and volunteerism, 102
Case studies, persons with AIDS and
      substance abuse, group work
      with, 35, 36-37, 39-51
Cerney, M.S., 125, 127, 130
Chat group, 144
Child and Family Services Act (1984),
   185-186
Child factors, adoption disruption, 195
Child molester ("diddler"), 78
Childhood sex abuse, 77

Children, with mentally ill parents. *See*
      Mentally ill parents, group
      intervention with
Children's Aid Society (New York
      City), 148, 150, 151, 162. *See
      also* Families for
      Reunification: Partners in the
      Plan
Children's group sessions, post–legal
      adoption families, 199-201
Clary, E., 102, 105, 122
Cohen, J.S., 195
Cohler, B., 177
Collaboration, groups as opportunity
      for, 160-161
Competency-led group approach, 55
Comprehensive biopsychosocial
      assessment, 79
Confidentiality, 185
Conrad, D., 103
Consensual validation, group field
      instruction, 62
Constructive confrontation, 81
Consumer satisfaction questionnaire,
      157-158
Consumer-based approach, 186
Contemplative stage, 28
Context, and volunteerism, 101
Contingency plan, 186
Cooperation, degree of, 172, 173
Core group, 178
Counselling, families of organ donors,
      116
Counterpersonal, 37
Coverdale, J., 170
Cowbum, M., 55
Cowger, C.D., 149
Craig-Oldsen, H.L., 150
Credibility, moderator, 123-126
Cross-cultural service learning, 103
Cross-national encounter, 17-19
Cross-talk, 33
Cultural encounter, constructing a, 22f
Cultural isolation, 138-139
Culturocentrism, 19

Curriculum, group work with
    post–legal adoption families,
    199-204

Daly, M., 120
Davies, L.J., 195
Deference, process of, 16
"Demand for work," 42
Denial, 173
Denver Mother's and Children's
    Project, 176-177
Department of Health and Human
    Services, 193
Devotions Upon Emergent Occasions
    (Donne), 95
Dialogue, group as opportunity for,
    160-161
DiClemente, C.C., 28
Disease model, alcohol, 31
Dixon, L., 182
Donne, John, 95
Douglass, G.E., 120
"Drunkalogue," 33

Écoumène, humanizing or idealizing, 6
Educational group, 142, 143, 184
Emic, 19
Emotions, normalization of, 127-128
Empathic demand for work, 39
Empathy, victim, 90-91
Empowerment praxis, 134
Entry group, 178
Epstein, L., 150
Erikson, E., 108
Etic, 19
Exclusion, process of, 57

"Facilitation" style, group work, 56
Facilitative confrontation, 42
Faculty liaison role, field education,
    62-64, 70
Faculty orientation, 65
Faha, G., 63
Falck, H., 169

Families for Reunification: Partners in
    the Plan
    analysis of, 157-162
    assessment of, 162-164
    program design, 152-156
Family reunification goals, 91-92
Father, mentally ill, 184-185. *See also*
    Mentally ill parents, group
    intervention with
Feedback
    group field instruction, 62
    post–legal adoption families,
    204-206
Fein, E., 195
Female cotherapist, role of, 87-90
"Female culture," 11-12
Female perspective, 88-89
Fidele, N., 44
Field placement, service education,
    104-107
Field-consulting function, faculty
    liaison, 63, 70
Field-consulting
    methodology/outcomes, 70-72
"Fifteen Skills for Managing
    Behavior," MAPP/GPS
    program, 156
"Fight-or-flight" syndrome, 37, 41
First names, moderator use of, 124
Focus groups, 115-117, 142, 143
    for Asian women, 137-138. *See also*
    Asian mothers' support
    project, research and action
    beginning, 129
    and emotions, normalization of,
    127-128
    group members' self disclosure,
    126-127
    moderator self-disclosure and
    credibility, 123-126
    participants, motivation of, 122-123
    participants' comments,
    legitimization of, 128-129
    and the screener questionnaire,
    119-122
    and sensitive topics, 117-119

Follow-up support, families of organ donors, 116
lack of, 120
Formation stage, 32-35
Fortune, A., 63
Functional group work models, 150
Functional School, 84
Fund-raising, 106

Garvin, C., 150, 169, 173
Gender, 11-12, 13
Gender roles, spouses of international students, 139
Germain, C., 149, 168
Getzel, G.S., 60, 61
Gildner, M., 155, 156
Gitterman, A., 61, 149, 168
Glassman, U., 61, 62
Globalisation, 5
"Go-between," social worker as, 8
Goldberg, J.R., 60
Goldman, J., 181
Goodman, S., 178
Googins, B., 29-30
Gopfert, M., 172
Great Britain, group work in, 53-57
Greif, G.L., 32
Grounding, 86-87
Group (G), 17
definition of, 168-170
identification with, 102
purpose of, 33
synergy through, 142-144
"Group as life," 175
"Group citizens," 80, 81, 93-94
Group dependent, 82
Group field consulting, 59
faculty liaison role, 62-64, 70
group progress reviews, 67-68
group supervision models, 61-62
individual tutorial models, 60
methodology, 70-72
multicomponent models, 60-61
orientations, 64-65

Group field consulting *(continued)*
outcomes, 70-72
student integration seminars, 65-66, 71
Group field-consulting model, 64-68, 69
Group intervention model
male sex offenders, 75
and mentally ill parents, 174-181
Group manual, 203
Group members' self-disclosure, 126-127
Group modality, 180
Group Preparation and Selection process, 150
Group progress review, 67-68
Group services, 198-199
Group supervision models, 61-62
Group work
and alliances, creation of, 1-2
birth parent self-assessment, 147-149
Families for Reunification: Partners in the Plan, 152-164
MAPP/GPS, development of, 149-152
in Great Britain, 53-57
group field consulting, 59
faculty liaison role, 62-64, 70
group progress reviews, 67-68
group supervision models, 61-62
individual tutorial models, 60
methodology, 70-72
multicomponent models, 60-61
outcomes, 70-72
orientations, 64-65
student integration seminars, 65-66, 71
international
and the cross-national encounter, 17-19
"inter" to "trans"-cultural, 19-24
and the "magic square," 14, 15f
and politeness, 15-16
and self-centered learning, 16
and women-only groups, 16-17

Group work *(continued)*
  with male sex offenders, 75-76
    comprehensive biopsychological
      assessment, 79
    and family reunification goals,
      91-92
    and female cotherapists, role of,
      87-90
    and the good group citizen role,
      93-94
    and grounding, 86-87
    "here and now and everyday life"
      issues, addressing, 85-86
    integration of new group
      members, 93
    marginalized, 92-93
    pretherapy psychoeducation,
      79-80
    psychosocial focal group therapy,
      80-81
    and resocialization, 92-93
    societal control versus self-
      control, 83-85
    supervised mutual aid and
      interactional therapy, 82-83
    the tortured souls, 76-79
    unstructured dynamic group
      therapy, 81
    as victims, 90-91
  with mentally ill parents, 167-168
    definition of, 168-170
    difficulties with, 172-174
    features of, 171-172
    implications of, 181-187
    prevalence of, 170-171
    studies, 175-181
  with persons with AIDS
    recovering from substance
      abuse, 27-29
    authority theme, 35-37
    case studies, 35, 36-37, 38-51
    formation stage, 32-35
    intimacy theme, 37-51
  with post–legal adoption families,
    group work with, 193-194
    adoption disruption, 194-196

Group work, with post–legal adoption
  families, group work with
  (continued)
    curriculum, 199-204
    group services, 198-199
    importance of, 197-198
    outcome evaluation, 204-206
    population studied, 196-197
    program design, 199
  for research and action, Asian
    mothers' support project,
    133-134
    cultural isolation, 138-139
    focus groups, 137-138
    gender roles, 139
    North Campus Outreach Project
      (NCOP), 134-137
    programming, 139-140
    results, 141-142
    structural difficulties, 139
    survey and program data,
      140-141
    and synergy through groups,
      142-144
  in service education, 99-100
    effects of group work
      intervention, 107-111
    field placement, 104-107
    future of, 111-112
    levels of transcendence identified
      in group interaction, 112-113
    "Making a River," poem,
      110-111
    volunteerism, reasons for,
      102-103
  teleconferencing focus groups,
    115-117
    beginning, 129
    and emotions, normalization of,
      127-128
    group members' self disclosure,
      126-127
    moderator self-disclosure and
      credibility, 123-126
    participants, motivation of,
      122-123

Group work, teleconferencing focus groups *(continued)*
 participants' comments, legitimization of, 128-129
 and the screener questionnaire, 119-122
 and sensitive topics, 117-119
Group work intervention, effects of, 107-111
Grunebaum, H., 179, 182

Hall, Toynbee, 85, 100
Hardesty, L., 32
Hard-to-place children, study of, 195
Hartman, A., 197-198
Hassles Scale, 141
Hedin, D., 103
Helper principle, 102
Henderson Hospital program, 180
Hepworth, D.H., 149
"Here and now and everyday life," 85-86
Hess, P.M., 156
Hofstede, G., 9
Home Care Program, 177-178
Home group/nation (HG), 17-19
Home visit program, 179
Homogenisation, of culture, 6
Hornby, H., 197
Hull House, Chicago, 100

Identification with group, 102
Identify resources in the community, Families for Reunification group session nine, 154, 163, 164
Identity, Youth and Crisis (Erikson), 108
Identity development, and community service, 104, 108
IDIG (international development of international group work), 8
Incest, 77

Individual tutorial models, 60
Individuality, 10-11, 13
Informational myths, 30
Initiation process, female cotherapist, 88
"Insider-outsider" debate, 19
Integration of new group members, 93
Intensive model, fieldwork, 63
"Inter" to "trans"-cultural, 19-24
Interactional therapy, 82-83
Interdependence, value of, 82-83
International group work, 8-13
 and the cross-national encounter, 17-19
 "inter" to "trans"-cultural, 19-24
 and the "magic square," 14, 15f
 and politeness, 15-16
 and self-centered learning, 16
 and women-only groups, 16-17
International relationship arc, 23f
International students. *See* Asian mothers' support project, research and action
Internet, 5
Interpersonal skills, lack of, 172, 173
Intimacy theme, 37-51
Isolation, 172-173

Jenkins, A., 176
Journal writing, 66
Justice, and levels of transcendence, 113

Kaplan, T., 62
Kimberley, M.D., 76, 79
Kisthardt, W.E., 149
Knight, G., 195
Know your family, Families for Reunification group session two, 152, 162, 163
Know your rights, Families for Reunification group session one, 152, 162, 163

Konopka, G., 55
Kübler-Ross, Elisabeth, 155, 156
Kurland, R., 169

Lang, N., 175, 183
Larsen, J.A., 149
Lee, J., 188
Legitimisation of participants'
    comments, 119, 128-129
Lehman, A., 182
Lifelong vulnerability philosophy,
    82-83
"Linkage" function, 62
Lucas, L., 179
Lyons-Roth, K., 179, 182

"Magic square," 14, 15f
Maintain a safe and healthy home,
    Families for Reunification
    group session eight, 153-154,
    163, 164
"Making a river," poem, 110-111
Maladaptive defense, 42
"Male culture," 11-12
Male sex offenders, 75-76
    comprehensive biopsychological
        assessment, 79
    and family reunification goals,
        91-92
    and female cotherapists, role of,
        87-90
    and the good group citizen role,
        93-94
    and grounding, 86-87
    "here and now and everyday life"
        issues, addressing, 85-86
    integration of new group members,
        93
    marginalized, 92-93
    pretherapy psychoeducation, 79-80
    psychosocial focal group therapy,
        80-81
    and resocialization, 92-93

Male sex offenders *(continued)*
    societal control versus self-control,
        83-85
    supervised mutual aid and
        interactional therapy, 82-83
    the tortured souls, 76-79
    unstructured dynamic group
        therapy, 81
    as victims, 90-91
Manage children's behavior, Families
    for Reunification group
    session six, 153, 163, 164
MAPP, 148
MAPP/GPS program, 148-152
MAPP Group Preparation and
    Selection (MAPP/GPS)
    program, 148-152
Marital relationships and mental illness,
    171
Marshack., E., 60-61, 62
Marywood University, 99. *See also*
    Service education
Matano, R.A., 31
Matorin, S., 69
McDonald, T., 197
Mediating model for group work
    design, 159f
Memorial University Program, 79
Mentally ill parents, group intervention
    with, 167-168
    definition of, 168-170
    difficulties with, 172-174
    features of, 171-172
    implications of, 181-187
    prevalence of, 170-171
    studies, 175-181
Meuser, K., 181
Middleman, R., 169, 188
Miller, I., 61
Model Approach to Partnerships in
    Parenting (MAPP), 148
Moderator self-disclosure, 119,
    123-126
Modi, P., 55
Mondialisation, 5, 6

Morally inferior, alcoholics labeled as, 30
Morrison, M.C., 84
Mother, mentally ill, 184-185. *See also* Mentally ill parents, group intervention with
Motivation, focus group participant, 122-123
Mowbray, C., 170, 180
Multicomponent models, 60-61
Multiculturalism, 2
Musik, J., 177
Mutual aid
   group, 142-143
   and group field instruction, 62, 65
   integrating continued therapy with supervised, 75-79
   supervised, 82-83
   with treated sex offenders, 83-94
   work with persons with AIDS, 33

Narcotics Anonymous (NA), 30
National Institute for Social Work, 56
Nationalism, 6
Nation-state, 7
Need statement, 162-164
New group members, integration of, 93
New York State Department of Social Services (NYSDSS), 148
NEWPIN (London, England), 175
Next Step Programme of the New South Wales (NSW) Red Cross Blood Transfusion Service (BTS), 120, 130
Nicholson, J., 180, 182, 186
Nikkel, R., 180
Norberg, W., 64
North Campus Outreach Project (NCOP), 134-137. *See also* Asian mothers' support project, research and action

Offender as victim, 90-91

One-to-one treatment, 55
Operationalized transcendence, 109
Orel, N., 102
Organ donation, focus group. *See* Teleconferencing focus groups
Organisational contacts, 17
Organizational group work models, 150
Orientations, students and faculty, 64-65
"Other"
   comparing one's fate with, 113
   as an ordinary person, 112
Other culture/nation (OC/N), 17-19
Outcome evaluation, 204-206
Overpersonal, 37

PACE Program, 178
PACT Program, 178
Page, R.C., 82
Papell, C., 167
Parent factors, adoption disruption, 195
Parent group sessions, post–legal adoption families, 202-203
Parents, mentally ill. *See* Mentally ill parents, group intervention with
Participants' comments, legitimization of, 128-129
Partridge, S., 197
Pearson, I.Y., 118
Pedophilia, 77, 84
Peer group support, 104, 108
Penn, D., 181
Perry, W.G., 103
Personality, and volunteerism, 101
Persons with AIDS and substance abuse, group work with, 27-29
   authority theme, 35-37
   case studies, 35, 36-37, 38-51
   formation stage, 32-35
   intimacy theme, 37-51
Person-to-person help, 33

Plasse, B.R., 155
Politeness, and international group
     work, 15-16
Political contacts, 17
Post–legal adoption families, group
     work with, 193-194
  adoption disruption, 194-196
  curriculum, 199-204
  group services, 198-199
  importance of, 197-198
  outcome evaluation, 204-206
  population studied, 196-197
  program design, 199
Power, and volunteerism, 102
Practice-based model building, 56
Preparation, focus group, 129
Pretherapy psychoeducation, 79-80
Problem swapping, 35
Problematising, 21
Proch, K.O., 156
Prochaska, J.O., 28
Program data, focus group, 140-141
Programming, focus group, 139-140
Project CHILD (Providence, RI), 175
Protective factors, and volunteerism,
     102
Psychodrama techniques, 87
Psychosocial focal group therapy,
     80-81
Psychosocial group work models, 150
Public perception, sex offenders, 76
"Pulling together," 83
Purcell, J., 182
Pyle, K., 103, 107

Racism, confronting, 57
Rank, Otto, 84
Regionalism, 6
Reid, W., 150
Rejection
  family, 91
  promoting, 88
Relapse, 45-51
  prevention, 80

Relational theory, 44
Relative hierarchical distance (RHD),
     9-10, 13
Reoffending, risk of, 83
Research and action, Asian mothers'
     support project, 133-134
  cultural isolation, 138-139
  focus groups, 137-138
  gender roles, 139
  North Campus Outreach Project
     (NCOP), 134-137
  programming, 139-140
  results, 141-142
  structural difficulties, 139
  survey and program data, 140-141
  and synergy through groups,
     142-144
Research-action program, 7
Resocialization, male sex offenders,
     92-93
Resonance, 44
Responsibility, and levels of
     transcendence, 113
Reunification goals, family, 91-92
Reynolds, Bertha, 61
Ridge, R., 102, 105, 122
Risk taking, 12-13
Rubovits, P., 175
Rogosch, F., 170, 180
Rowe, W., 76, 79

Saleebey, D., 147-148, 149, 158, 159,
     161
Salmon, R., 60, 61, 169
Schields, G., 102
Schizophrenia, 170, 174. *See also*
     Mentally ill parents, group
     intervention with
Schneck, C., 64
Schneck, D., 63
Schondel, C., 102
Schroeder, H., 181
Schwartz, W., 42, 149, 158, 159,
     168-169

Screener questionnaire, reactivity to,
    119-122
Seeman, M., 167-168, 170, 180
Selecting in, 150, 151
Selecting out, 151
Self-actualization, 85
Self-assessment, birth parent, 147-149
    Families for Reunification: Partners
        in the Plan, 152-164
    MAPP/GPS, development of,
        149-152
Self-centered learning, 16
Self-disclosure
    group members', 126-127
    moderator, 119, 123-126
Self-esteem, 102
Self-help groups
    alcoholism, 30
    post–legal adoption families, 199
    and synergy, 142, 143-144
Self-monitoring philosophy, 82-83, 84
Self-rebuilding, 76
Self-serving, 102
Semistructured group therapy, 80
Sensitive topics, and teleconferencing
        focus groups, 117-119
Service education, 99-100
    effects of group work intervention,
        107-111
    field placement, 104-107
    future of, 111-112
    levels of transcendence identified in
        group interaction, 112-113
    "Making a River," poem, 110-111
    volunteerism, reasons for, 102-103
Settlement house movement, 100
Sex offense history, 77
Sexism, confronting, 57
Sexual abuse, by females, 89-90
Sexual decision making, focus groups
        for, 119
Sexual dynamics, female cotherapist,
        89
Sexual victimization patterns, 77-78
Shamdasani, P.N., 115-117, 122
Sheppard, H.A., 37

Shulman, L., 82, 90
Singular gatekeeper, 69
Smith, D.H., 101
Smith, H.Y., 63
Snyder, M., 102, 105, 122
Social background, and volunteerism,
        101
Social exclusion, fight against, 56
Social factor, and volunteerism, 102
Social subsidiarity, 7
Social work, supervision and field
        instruction in
    and faculty liaison, 62-64, 70
    group supervision models, 61-62
    individual tutorial models, 60
    multicomponent models, 60-61
Socialization, into professional role, 66
Societal control versus self-control,
        83-85
Societal norms, and focus groups, 125
Solidarity, process of, 16
Spouse, of international student, 135.
        See also Asian mothers'
        support project, research and
        action
Spring Break Service trips, Appalachia,
        99, 105. *See also* Service
        education
St. Louis model, group care, 180
Statutory responsibilities, 53-54
Stewart, D.W., 115-117, 122
Stott, F., 177
Stress, and cultural isolation, 138-139
Structural difficulties, spouses of
        international students, 139
Student development, measuring,
        103-104
Student integration seminars, 65-66, 71
Student orientation, 64-65
Substance abuse and persons with
        AIDS, group work with,
        27-29
    authority theme, 35-37
    case studies, 35, 36-37, 38-51
    formation stage, 32-35
    intimacy theme, 37-51

Sudden loss, understanding, 118
Supervision, and field instruction
  definition of, 69
  and faculty liaison, 62-64, 70
  group supervision models, 61-62
  individual tutorial models, 60
  multicomponent models, 60-61
Supervisory components, 60
Survey, focus group, 140-141
Synergy, through groups, 142-144, 160

Task group, 142, 143
Teen group sessions, post–legal
      adoption families, 201-202
Teleconferencing focus groups,
      115-117
  beginning, 129
  and emotions, normalization of,
      127-128
  group members' self disclosure,
      126-127
  moderator self-disclosure and
      credibility, 123-126
  participants, motivation of, 122-123
  participants' comments,
      legitimization of, 128-129
  and the screener questionnaire,
      119-122
  and sensitive topics, 117-119
Termination
  adoption, 194-196. *See also*
      Post–legal adoption families,
      group work with
  client, 66, 82
Third level group project, 75-76
Threshold Psychosocial Program,
      177-178
Through-care service, 57
Tortured souls, 76-79
Toynbee Hall, 100
Transcendence development, 104,
      112-113
Transgender female, Tania, 34

Translation, process of, 21-22
Treating the treated, 79-83
Tremitiere, B.T., 195
Trouble-shooting model, fieldwork, 63
Tuckman, B., 14
Twelve-step models, use of, 30

Übersetzen (to translate), 22
Understanding, and volunteerism, 102
Universalism, 6
"University of hard knocks," 87
University of Kansas School of Social
      Work, 149
University of Michigan, 133. *See also*
      Asian mothers' support
      project, research and action
Unstructured dynamic group therapy, 81
Unstructured therapeutic process
      model, 81

Value-bearing institutions, 108
Values, 56
  and volunteerism, 102
Volunteerism. *See* Service education

Waldo, M., 180
Watson, K., 198
"We group," 19
Webster, J., 172
Welfare state, 7-8
Westhus, A., 195
Woman-only group, 16-17
Wood, G., 169
Wright Mills, C., 20

Yalom, I.D., 31
Yates, M., 104, 108, 109
  "The year of the feelings," 28
Youniss, J., 104, 108, 109
YWCA movement, 85

Zeller, R.A.
  and emotions, normalization of, 128
  and moderators' self-disclosure and
      credibility, 123-124, 126
  and participants' comments,
      legitimization of, 128
  and sexual decision making, focus
      groups for, 119
  and reactivity to screener
      questionnaire, 119-120,
      121-122
Zemencuk, J., 170